100+ Funny Short Stories for Seniors

Large Print, Easy-to-Read Tales of Laughter and Joy — A Funny Gift for Retirement, Birthday, Father's Day, Mother's Day and More

Edward Harper

Table of Contents

About me and Why I Wrote This Book 5
Borrowed Glasses, Blurry Day 6
When the Shopping List Goes Wrong 7
Grandma vs. the Remote 8
Mismatched Shoes, Perfect Night 9
Keys on Ice 10
Stranger Chat in the Elevator 11
Whose Coat Is This Anyway? 12
The Ringing Purse Mystery 13
Car Twins in the Parking Lot 14
The Whisper Everyone Heard 15
Switched Birthday Cakes 16
Grandkids' Magic Tricks Gone Wild 17
Grandma Opens the Wrong Gift 18
Family Portrait Mayhem 19
Who Sits Where at Thanksgiving? 20
The Joke That Made No Sense 21
Grandma's Recipe Hiding in the Bills 22
A Cat at the Dinner Table 23
Grandpa, the Generous Tooth Fairy 24
When the Picnic Blanket Took Off 25
Breakfast with the Smoke Alarm 26
Soda Pop Shower 27
Too Hot to Handle Soup 28
Coffee Everywhere but the Cup 29
Grandpa, the Cookie Thief 30
Spaghetti Stuck Together 31
A Teakettle with a Tune 32
When Sugar Tasted Salty 33
Catch That Shopping Cart! 34
The Day the Pie Deflated 35
Auto-Correct Strikes Again 36
Frozen Face on Video Chat 37

Searching for the Wi-Fi Code 38
The Lost with the GPS 39
Oops, Wrong Inbox... 40
Selfie Stick Shenanigans 41
Roomba vs. the Cat 42
The Package That Wasn't Right 43
The Alarm Clock That Didn't Stop... 44
Alexa, What Did You Just Do? 45
Sausage Thief on Four Legs 46
Yarn Basket Cat Nap... 47
Parrot Playing Telephone 48
Hamster on the Loose... 49
Goldfish with a Starring Role 50
Best Friends: Dog and Postman 51
Neighborhood Watch Cat 52
Goat in the Living Room 53
Picnic Basket Stowaway.. 54
Bus-Riding Cat...55
The Man with the Crooked Hat 56
Sing-Along on the City Bus..57
Sitting in the Wrong Row 58
Umbrellas Dancing in the Parade.. 59
Pumpkins That Weren't for Dinner 60
Melting Ice Cream Mayhem 61
The Suitcase That Refused to Follow.. 62
Comedians on the Park Bench 63
The Wrong Bus Ticket 64
The Seaside Sandcastle Collapse 65
Singing the Wrong Words 66
Slip on Stage at the Talent Show 67
The Camping Tent Collapse 68
Tangled Up in Fishing Lines 69
Costume Fail at the Party 70
When April Fools Backfires 71
Salt Instead of Sugar...72

Shopping List for Homework 73
The Neighborhood Parade Giggle.. 74
Singing with the Frogs 75
The Hearing Aid Surprise 76
Calling the Wrong Old Friend 77
Dentures on the Loose 78
Chasing the Runaway Cane 79
Sock Skating in the Hallway 80
Looking for Glasses Already Worn 81
Bingo Numbers All Wrong... 82
Two Trips, Same Shopping List 83
Wallet Found in the Freezer 84
Lost but Laughing on the Road 85
Christmas Lights in a Knot 86
The Turkey That Wouldn't Fit the Oven 87
Valentine's Card to the Wrong Man 88
Melted Chocolate Egg Hunt 89
Little Firework with Big Sparks 90
Twins in the Same Costume 91
Celebrating Midnight Too Early 92
Runaway Birthday Balloons 93
Sweaters That Didn't Fit Anyone... 94
Carols Sung with Made-Up Lyrics 95
The Church Potluck Mystery Dish 96
Talent Show Gone Off Script 97
When Nobody Agreed on the Rules 98
Sold by Mistake at the Yard Sale 99
Laugh Attack at Choir Practice 100
Who Really Won the Raffle?...101
Cookies Without Sugar 102
Spray Battle in the Garden 103
Dancing Contest in the Street 104
The Couch Stuck in the Doorway...105
The Midnight Train Song... 106
Did These Stories Make You Smile? 107

About me and Why I Wrote This Book

Hello! I'd like to share a little about myself and what led me to create this book.

I've always believed that laughter is one of life's simplest and most powerful gifts. A good chuckle has the ability to ease tension, lift our spirits, and remind us not to take ourselves too seriously. Over the years, I've noticed how the funniest moments are often the smallest ones—burning the toast, mixing up names, or watching a family pet steal the spotlight. These are the kinds of everyday mishaps that bring people together, turning ordinary days into memories worth retelling.

That belief is what inspired this collection. I wanted to gather lighthearted, easy-to-read stories that shine a spotlight on the humor we can find in daily life. While so many books focus on nostalgia and reflection, I felt there was also room for a collection that simply makes us laugh.

I dedicated this book to seniors because laughter truly has no age limit. In fact, I think it becomes even more precious as the years go by. Sharing a funny story with a friend, a grandchild, or even just enjoying it quietly with a cup of tea can make the day brighter.

My hope is that these stories bring you genuine smiles, a sense of lightness, and maybe even spark a memory of your own funny moments worth sharing. If this book gives you a reason to laugh out loud—or better yet, laugh together with someone you love—then it has fulfilled its purpose.

With warmth and a smile,

Edward

Borrowed Glasses, Blurry Day

Arthur prided himself on his morning routine. Every day, he shuffled into the kitchen, poured a steaming cup of coffee, and sat down to read the newspaper before his wife, Margaret, joined him. On this particular morning, though, something seemed off. The print on the page swam in front of his eyes, letters blurring into a rainbow haze. He rubbed his temples and muttered, "Must be getting old."

Margaret breezed in, humming as she prepared her tea. Arthur squinted at her. She looked strangely glowing, her sweater a vivid pink that nearly blinded him. "Did you buy a new outfit?" he asked, tilting his head.

Margaret raised an eyebrow. "This? It's the same gray cardigan I've worn for years."

Arthur frowned. Later, when he turned on the television, the news anchor's face appeared tinted rose. Even the traffic lights outside seemed distorted, the red glaring like neon and the green a swampy blur. He muttered under his breath, "Either I'm losing my vision, or the whole world's been painted with watercolors."

Determined not to worry his wife, Arthur went about his day. At the grocery store, he leaned dangerously close to the labels, trying to distinguish "tomato soup" from "clam chowder." Shoppers gave him sympathetic looks as he squinted, mumbling about fonts being too small. Crossing the parking lot, he misread a stop sign, convinced it was octagonal but glowing purple. He laughed nervously to himself, shaking his head. "Maybe I should call the eye doctor."

When he returned home, Margaret was waiting with a grin. "Arthur," she said, holding out her hand, "what's this?" In her palm rested her reading glasses—sleek frames with tinted lenses she used only for knitting under bright light. Arthur touched his own face and froze. Sure enough, perched on his nose were Margaret's glasses, the culprit behind his day of kaleidoscopic vision.

Margaret burst out laughing, wiping tears from her eyes. "You've been wandering around town in my reading glasses all day! No wonder the world looked like a circus."

Arthur chuckled, relieved. "Well, it explains why the weatherman's suit looked like it belonged at a carnival." He carefully traded the tinted lenses for his own pair. The world snapped back into focus, crisp and ordinary once more. Still smiling, he reached for Margaret's hand. "I suppose it's good to see life through your eyes once in a while."

And she replied, still giggling, "Just don't make it a habit."

When the Shopping List Goes Wrong

Frank adored spending time with his grandchildren, though he often suspected they enjoyed playing little tricks on him. One Saturday morning, his daughter handed him a folded grocery list, hastily written by the kids. "Dad, would you mind picking these things up?"

Happy to help, Frank set off for the supermarket. The first item puzzled him: *marshmallows for salad*. He shrugged. "Must be some new recipe." Two bags went into the cart.

Next came *banana shampoo*. Frank squinted at the paper. "Shampoo made from bananas?" In the hair care aisle, he found a yellow bottle with a banana on it. Perfect.

The list grew stranger. *Pickles for dessert. Chocolate spaghetti. Peanut butter candles.* Frank scratched his head but decided not to question the imagination of the younger generation. "They're always trying something new," he muttered, pushing his cart with confidence.

At checkout, the cashier raised an eyebrow at the odd assortment. "Planning a party?"

"Family dinner," Frank replied with a wink.

Back home, he unloaded his treasures. His daughter entered, stared, and burst out laughing. "Dad... what is all this?"

Frank handed her the list. She read it aloud, tears streaming with laughter. "They wrote this as a joke! Banana shampoo? Chocolate spaghetti? Oh, Dad..."

The children peeked around the doorway, giggling uncontrollably. "Did you get everything, Grandpa?"

Frank folded his arms, trying to look serious. "Of course. And tonight, we're having the weirdest dinner ever."

That evening, the family gathered around the table, sampling absurd combinations like marshmallows on lettuce and pickles dipped in chocolate syrup. Frank dramatically slurped "banana shampoo spaghetti" made from noodles and syrup.

"It's... surprisingly terrible," he announced, sending the kids into hysterics.

From then on, Grandpa's grocery list disaster was retold at every gathering, always ending in laughter.

Grandma vs. the Remote

Evelyn liked to think she was up to date with technology. After all, she had learned how to text her grandchildren and even joined their weekly video calls. But one quiet afternoon, she faced a battle she hadn't expected: the television remote. Settling into her armchair, she aimed at the TV and pressed the buttons. Nothing happened. She pressed harder, jabbing at the arrows and the channel numbers. "This thing's useless," she muttered, shaking it like a stubborn ketchup bottle.

Frustrated, she marched into the kitchen. "Harold!" she called to her husband. "The remote is broken again."

Harold ambled in, adjusting his glasses. "Let me see." Evelyn handed him the device. He frowned, turned it over, and chuckled. "Evie, this isn't the remote. It's the cordless phone." Evelyn blinked, then looked down at the object in her hand. Sure enough, there were numbers, a receiver button, and even a blinking voicemail light. She gasped, then covered her face with both hands. "Oh no. I've been trying to change the channel with the phone."

Her grandchildren, who had just arrived for a visit, burst into laughter. "Grandma, did you try to call the TV?" one teased.

Evelyn laughed along, her cheeks warm with embarrassment. "Well, I gave it my best shot. At least the TV didn't answer." That evening, after everyone had gone to bed, Evelyn sat alone with her tea. She looked at the phone and then at the remote, both sitting side by side on the table. With a mischievous smile, she picked up the phone, pointed it at the television, and said in her most commanding voice, "Channel seven, please."

The TV stayed silent, of course. But just then Harold's voice came from the kitchen: "Coming right up!" He shuffled in, changed the channel himself, and winked. Evelyn burst out laughing.

From then on, she liked to joke that she *did* have voice control—only it worked through Harold.

Mismatched Shoes, Perfect Night

George had never been much of a fashion enthusiast. Comfort always came before style, and if something matched, it was usually by accident. One Saturday evening, he was invited to a neighborhood birthday party. He put on his best shirt, combed his thinning hair, and slipped into what he thought were his usual black dress shoes.

At the party, he greeted everyone with his usual cheerful grin. People glanced at him with curious expressions, but George assumed it was because of his dazzling smile. It wasn't until he walked across the living room that a teenager pointed and whispered, "Check out his shoes!"

George looked down and froze. On his left foot was a polished black dress shoe. On his right, a faded brown loafer. The two didn't match at all. "Oh dear," he muttered, feeling his ears grow warm.

Before he could explain himself, the host clapped him on the shoulder. "Now that's bold, George! Mixing styles. I like it." Others chimed in, calling it "trendy" and "eccentric." Soon the mismatched shoes were the talk of the evening.

George, at first mortified, decided to play along. He struck a mock model pose, sticking one foot out dramatically. "They call this look 'Half Past Formal, Half Past Nap Time,'" he announced. Laughter rippled through the room.

As the night went on, people kept asking for photos with him. "Stand next to me, George," someone said, "I want proof that I was at the party with the man who set a new fashion trend." Even the DJ joined in, dedicating a song to "the man with the unforgettable shoes."

By the end of the evening, George was no longer embarrassed. He leaned over to a friend and whispered, "Maybe I should wear different shoes more often. No one will ever forget me now."

The next morning, when he told his wife about the accident, she laughed until tears rolled down her cheeks. "George, you may have started a neighborhood tradition."

And perhaps he did. Because from then on, whenever someone wanted to add a little humor to a party, they showed up in mismatched shoes—an unspoken tribute to George and his unforgettable fashion statement.

Keys on Ice

Martha prided herself on being organized. Her keys were always placed in the little ceramic dish by the front door, right where they belonged. So when she was ready to head out for her morning walk and the dish was empty, she froze in disbelief.

"They must have slipped under the mail," she muttered, rifling through envelopes. Nothing. She patted her coat pockets, her handbag, even the cardigan she hadn't worn in days. Still no keys.

Her husband, Charles, looked up from his newspaper. "Lose something again?" he teased.

"Not again," Martha replied firmly. "They've simply misplaced themselves."

The hunt began. Couch cushions, rug, curtains—nothing. Charles peeked in the breadbox, chuckling, "Maybe you put them in with the toast."

An hour later, Martha sighed and opened the fridge for a drink—only to find her keyring gleaming beside the milk. "Charles! Come see this!"

He nearly doubled over laughing. "Well, at least they stayed nice and cool."

The next morning, when Martha grabbed yogurt from the fridge, she spotted the TV remote tucked between the grapes. She turned to Charles, who sipped his coffee innocently.

"Really?" she asked.

He grinned. "Just keeping you sharp."

From then on, the refrigerator became the family's unofficial lost-and-found—sometimes by accident, sometimes by design.

Stranger Chat in the Elevator

Harold considered himself a friendly man. He believed every elevator ride was an opportunity to brighten someone's day with a little conversation. So when he stepped into the elevator one Tuesday morning and saw a man about his age, Harold's face lit up.

"Well, if it isn't Jerry!" he exclaimed, clapping the stranger on the shoulder. "Haven't seen you since the fishing trip. How's that old boat of yours holding up?"

The man blinked in confusion. "Uh... excuse me?"

Harold chuckled. "Still the same jokester, I see. Remember when you almost fell in trying to catch that trout? Classic Jerry!"

The stranger gave a polite but baffled smile. "I think you might have me confused with someone else."

Harold waved the comment away. "Don't be modest. How's your wife doing? What was her name again... Patricia?"

The man shifted uncomfortably, gripping his briefcase. "My wife's name is Linda. And I've never owned a boat."

The elevator doors opened at the next floor, but Harold kept talking as though nothing was amiss. "Linda, Patricia, close enough. Tell her I said hello!"

By now, the stranger was chuckling despite himself. "Sir, I promise you, I'm not Jerry." There was a pause. Harold squinted, finally taking a good look. His eyes widened. "Well, I'll be... you're right. You're not Jerry." Then he burst out laughing, clutching his stomach. "You look *just like him!* I've been carrying on like an old fool."

The stranger laughed too, shaking his head. "Well, at least you made this elevator ride more interesting."

When the doors opened again, they stepped out together, still chuckling. Harold extended his hand. "Since you're not Jerry, I suppose we should start fresh. I'm Harold."

"Nice to meet you, Harold. I'm Tom," the man replied with a grin.

From that day forward, whenever Harold saw Tom in the lobby, he'd wink and say, "Morning, Jerry!" and Tom would laugh, replying, "Evening, Harold!"

What started as a case of mistaken identity turned into a genuine friendship, all thanks to an elevator ride and Harold's unshakable determination to make small talk.

Whose Coat Is This Anyway?

It had been a chilly evening, and Walter was eager to enjoy dinner at his favorite Italian restaurant. He hung his heavy wool coat on the rack near the entrance, patting the pocket to be sure his wallet was safe. With that done, he joined his friends at the table, ready for a night of pasta, laughter, and good company.

Hours later, with bellies full and spirits high, Walter returned to the coat rack. He slipped his arms into what he was certain was his own coat and strolled toward the door. It felt heavier than usual, but he ignored the thought and kept walking.

At home, as he emptied the pockets, the mystery began. Instead of his keys, he found a bright red scarf, a pair of leather gloves much too small for his hands, and a folded envelope with the words *For My Darling* written across it. Walter raised an eyebrow. Inside was a love letter, sweet and heartfelt, clearly meant for someone else. He chuckled to himself. "Well, I've brought home more than leftovers tonight."

The next day, he returned to the restaurant carrying the coat and its mysterious contents. Near the entrance stood another gentleman, holding Walter's wool coat. Their eyes met, and both men burst into laughter.

"I believe this belongs to you," the stranger said, handing over Walter's coat.

"And I think this one is yours," Walter replied, returning the red-scarfed coat. "I promise I didn't try on the gloves."

The man laughed, clearly relieved. "And my wife will be happy to know her letter found its way back safely."

As they shook hands, Walter smiled. The mix-up had turned into more than a funny anecdote. It was the kind of accident that might lead to a new friendship, and perhaps even a running joke whenever they crossed paths again.

The Ringing Purse Mystery

Clara loved her morning ritual at the little café on the corner. She would order a cappuccino, settle by the window, and watch the bustle of the street while enjoying the warmth of her drink. On one particular morning, however, her peaceful routine was interrupted by the sound of a phone ringing.

At first, she barely noticed. But the ringtone, a shrill tune, kept playing over and over. Clara glanced around the café, expecting someone to grab their phone. No one did. People shifted in their seats, whispering and rolling their eyes, but the ringing continued.

"It must belong to that man near the counter," Clara thought, watching a gentleman fiddling with his newspaper. When he did not move, she grew irritated. The ringing started again, echoing across the café. Clara sighed, leaned toward him, and said, "Sir, could you please answer your phone?"

The man looked up in surprise. "My phone? It hasn't rung once."

Another burst of the ringtone filled the air. Clara scanned the room, her annoyance growing. "Honestly, who leaves their phone on like this?" she muttered, shaking her head.

The sound seemed to follow her as she reached for her bag. She froze. The ringing was louder now, vibrating against her hand. With a sheepish expression, she dug into her purse and pulled out her own phone, which was lighting up with an incoming call.

The entire café chuckled. Clara's cheeks flushed crimson. "Oh dear... it was me all along." A young woman at the next table grinned. "At least your phone has good taste in making an entrance."

Clara laughed, embarrassed but amused. "I suppose my purse was too full to notice." She answered the call quickly, then slipped the phone back with a smile.

For the rest of the morning, customers exchanged knowing glances with her, and Clara found herself laughing every time she thought about it. What began as a small frustration turned into a shared moment of humor among strangers.

From that day forward, Clara always checked her bag before blaming anyone else. And every time she returned to the café, the barista teased, "Your phone behaving today, Clara?"

She would smile, hold up her bag, and reply, "Quiet as a mouse."

Car Twins in the Parking Lot

It was a sunny Saturday afternoon when Martin left the grocery store with a bag full of snacks and drinks. He strolled into the crowded parking lot, pressing the button on his car's key fob. A pair of headlights blinked in the distance, and he walked toward them with confidence.

At the same time, a woman named Linda was walking in from the other direction, also pressing her key fob. To her surprise, the very same car lit up and beeped. She quickened her pace.

Martin reached the car first and tugged at the handle, but the door refused to open. He frowned, pressing the button again. The lights blinked, but the door remained stubbornly locked.

On the other side, Linda was trying too. Her remote beeped, the car responded, and she yanked at the handle. Confused, the two of them looked up at the exact same moment, each staring across the roof of the identical vehicle.

"Excuse me," Martin said with a nervous laugh, "is this... your car?"

"I was about to ask you the same thing," Linda replied, equally bewildered.

They both stepped back and looked around. To their amazement, parked just one row over was another car, the same make, model, and even color. Martin pressed his fob again, and the other car flashed its lights. Linda tried hers, and sure enough, the car beside it beeped in response.

The two of them burst out laughing. "I thought my key was broken," Martin admitted.

"And I thought I had forgotten how to open a door," Linda said, still laughing.

Other shoppers glanced their way, amused by the scene. One man pushing a cart called out, "Happens more often than you'd think!"

Finally, Martin and Linda walked to their rightful cars, still chuckling. Before leaving, Martin leaned out the window. "Well, at least we know our cars have a twin."

Linda grinned and waved. "And maybe next time we'll remember where we parked before chasing the wrong one."

As they drove off in opposite directions, both were still smiling, knowing they would never forget the day they performed a little parking lot shuffle for an accidental audience.

The Whisper Everyone Heard

George loved his weekly trips to the library. He enjoyed the quiet atmosphere, the smell of books, and the chance to browse the shelves at his leisure. One afternoon, he spotted his friend Harold sitting at a table near the window. Excited to share a funny story, George tiptoed over and leaned down to whisper.

Only, it wasn't a whisper.

"Harold, you won't believe what my neighbor did with his lawnmower!" George boomed, his voice echoing through the hushed reading room.

Heads turned instantly. A woman near the dictionaries raised her eyebrows, while a student in the corner tried not to laugh. George continued, unaware of the scene he was causing. "He forgot to empty the bag and the thing sprayed grass clippings all over his laundry!"

Harold's face turned red, and he waved his hands frantically. "George, your hearing aid... it's on full volume."

George blinked in surprise. He reached to adjust the tiny device and realized Harold was right. He had been speaking far louder than he thought. Mortified, he looked around at the amused faces now staring at him.

For a brief moment, the library was silent again. Then the student in the corner let out a snicker, and soon the entire table of readers began chuckling. Even the stern-looking librarian walked over, her lips twitching as she tried to hide a smile.

"Mr. Thompson," she said kindly, "we encourage quiet voices in the library. But thank you for sharing such an entertaining story."

George's embarrassment melted into laughter. "Well, at least I gave everyone a break from studying," he replied.

Harold grinned. "Next time, just whisper into my good ear. Less risk of disturbing the entire library." As George settled into the chair across from him, he shook his head with a smile. "I suppose if I'm going to make an announcement, it should at least be something worth hearing."

The incident quickly became one of George's favorite tales to tell. Whenever he visited the library afterward, fellow patrons would greet him with a knowing smile.

And while he never quite mastered the art of whispering, George found comfort in the fact that sometimes, even in the quietest places, laughter could be the loudest sound of all.

Switched Birthday Cakes

The Johnsons and the Millers lived next door to each other and often shared little favors, from borrowing sugar to watering plants during vacations. One Saturday, both families were hosting birthday parties, one for little Lily who was turning five, and one for George, the grandfather who was celebrating his eightieth.

The local bakery had prepared two cakes. One was decorated with pink frosting, sprinkles, and big cheerful letters that read *Happy 5th, Lily!* The other was a stately chocolate cake with elegant white icing and the message *Happy 8oth, George*. Somewhere between the bakery and the front doors, the boxes were switched.

At the Johnson house, children gathered around the table, eyes wide with excitement as the cake was revealed. Instead of rainbows and unicorns, however, the words *Happy 8oth, George* stared back at them. For a moment, silence hung in the air. Then one little boy asked, "Who's George?" and the room erupted in giggles.

Next door, the Millers had their own surprise. George leaned forward, ready to blow out his candles, when his family unveiled a cake covered in pink frosting and candy flowers. The old man blinked, then laughed so hard he nearly lost his dentures. "I haven't been five in seventy-five years," he wheezed, wiping his eyes.

Soon the two families realized what had happened. Mrs. Johnson carried the chocolate cake next door while Mr. Miller brought the pink frosted one back. But instead of exchanging them quietly, everyone spilled into the yards, laughing and holding both cakes high.

"Why not celebrate together?" someone suggested. Tables were pushed together, chairs were gathered, and the two parties merged into one. Children darted around with balloons while the adults clinked glasses. George sang happy birthday to Lily, and Lily proudly sang back to George.

By the end of the evening, no one could remember which cake belonged to which family. All that mattered was the laughter, the frosting smeared across happy faces, and the shared memory of a mix-up that turned two small gatherings into one unforgettable celebration.

From that day on, the Johnsons and Millers made it a tradition to host joint birthday parties. After all, one cake was sweet, but two cakes shared with neighbors and friends were even better.

Grandkids' Magic Tricks Gone Wild

On a rainy Saturday afternoon, Evelyn and Robert's living room was transformed into a grand theater. Their grandchildren had been practicing all week for what they proudly called *The Amazing Magic Show*. Chairs were lined up, a blanket was draped across two chairs to serve as a curtain, and the youngest grandson handed out tickets made from scraps of construction paper.

"Ladies and gentlemen," announced ten-year-old Max with dramatic flair, "prepare to be amazed!"

The show began with card tricks. Max shuffled the deck so vigorously that half the cards slipped from his hands and scattered across the carpet. "Ta-da!" he declared, pretending it was part of the act. His sister Sophie pulled a rabbit out of her hat, except the rabbit was a stuffed toy that got stuck halfway. She tugged until it popped free, nearly hitting Grandpa in the nose.

Next came the coin trick. Sophie slipped a coin into her pocket, intending to make it vanish, but then forgot which pocket it was in. She patted herself frantically until the audience of two burst into laughter.

The finale was supposed to be the disappearing scarf. Max whispered to his sister to distract the grandparents while he tucked the scarf under the couch cushion. Unfortunately, the scarf dangled out visibly, bright red against the beige sofa. Robert pointed with a grin, "I think the magic escaped early."

Instead of being discouraged, the children stood tall and bowed deeply. "Thank you, thank you! You've been a wonderful audience!"

Evelyn clapped enthusiastically, her eyes sparkling. "That was the best show I've ever seen."

Robert added, "I've been to Las Vegas, but nothing compares to this level of entertainment."

The children giggled, pleased with themselves. Then they handed out autographs written in crayon, insisting their grandparents keep them as souvenirs.

Later that evening, Evelyn taped one of the tickets to the refrigerator. "Front-row seats to the best magic show in town," she said proudly.

For years afterward, the family would laugh about that rainy afternoon when a handful of clumsy tricks created so much joy. The show may not have fooled anyone, but it worked real magic: filling the house with laughter and love.

Grandma Opens the Wrong Gift

At Margaret's birthday party, the living room was filled with colorful balloons, the scent of cake, and a mountain of gift bags stacked on the coffee table. She felt spoiled as friends and family gathered around, eager to see her open each present.

She reached for a cheerful blue bag decorated with silver stars. Pulling out the tissue paper, she expected perhaps a scarf or a box of chocolates. Instead, she found a pair of enormous men's socks, clearly several sizes too big for her feet.

The room went silent for a moment before someone chuckled. "Maybe it's a new fashion trend?"

Margaret held up the socks, dangling them in the air. "Well, I always did want to try clown school." The guests burst into laughter.

Reaching deeper into the bag, she discovered a large ceramic mug. Bold letters across the front declared, *World's Best Grandpa*. That sent the entire room into hysterics.

Margaret threw her head back, laughing until her eyes watered. "Well, ladies and gentlemen, it looks like I've been promoted. As of today, I am officially the best grandpa in town."

Just then, a flustered voice piped up from across the room. "Oh no, that was my bag!" It was her neighbor Alan, who had brought a gift for his brother's retirement party later that evening. The two bags must have been mixed up on the table.

The mistake only made the moment funnier. Margaret handed the socks and mug back, still chuckling. "You'd better guard these carefully, Alan. I was starting to get attached."

Alan apologized, but everyone reassured him that the accident had made the party even more memorable. To keep the joke alive, Margaret slipped one of the oversized socks onto her hand and raised it like a puppet. "Grandpa says thank you for the wonderful birthday wishes!"

The guests roared with laughter again, and the story of the wrong gift bag became the highlight of the evening.

Later, as she unwrapped her real presents, Margaret smiled and said, "You know, the socks and mug might not have been mine, but they were the best gifts of the night."

Family Portrait Mayhem

The Jenkins family had gathered for their annual reunion, a tradition that brought cousins, aunts, uncles and grandparents together from near and far. As always, the highlight of the day was the group photo on the front lawn.

"Everyone outside!" Aunt Linda called, clutching her camera. "Let's capture this memory before the sun goes down."

Herding thirty relatives into one frame was no small task. The taller cousins were shuffled to the back, the little ones plopped onto blankets in the front, and the grandparents were seated proudly in the center.

"Smile!" Linda shouted as she set the timer and dashed to join the group. Just as the shutter clicked, Uncle Bill sneezed so loudly that his eyes squeezed shut and his shoulders shook. In the next shot, Cousin Sarah blinked while little Joey stuck out his tongue. The family dog, determined not to be left out, leapt into Grandpa's lap at exactly the wrong moment.

By the third attempt, frustration had turned to laughter. "All right, everyone look at the camera this time!" Linda pleaded. But as she counted down, the baby began crying and two teenagers whispered jokes that set off giggles across the back row.

The fourth photo caught Grandma mid-yawn and Aunt Carol waving to a neighbor passing by. Each new picture seemed worse than the last.

Finally, Linda sighed and pressed the button again. This time nobody bothered to pose. The children leaned against their parents, Grandpa held the dog like a trophy, and people laughed naturally instead of forcing smiles.

When Linda checked the results later, she realized the last shot was the best of all. Faces were relaxed, eyes sparkled with amusement, and the messy joy of the moment was more beautiful than any perfect portrait.

At the end of the reunion, copies of that picture were printed and mailed to every family member. It became the one everyone framed, proudly displayed not for its perfection but for its honesty. Visitors who admired it always got the same explanation from Grandma, who would grin and say, "That's us. Untidy, noisy, and exactly how we like it."

Who Sits Where at Thanksgiving?

Thanksgiving at the Peterson house was always lively. With cousins running through the hallways, uncles carving the turkey, and the aroma of pumpkin pie drifting from the kitchen, the day felt warm and full of cheer. But this year, the biggest laugh came not from a joke, but from the dinner table itself.

As everyone gathered to eat, no one seemed to remember where they were supposed to sit. Grandma had set out place cards, but the children had decided earlier that it would be funny to rearrange them. The result was pure chaos.

Uncle Frank found himself squeezed into the tiny chair meant for six-year-old Emily. "Either I've grown or this chair has shrunk," he grumbled, while everyone chuckled. Emily, meanwhile, proudly climbed into his tall seat, her feet dangling high above the floor.

Across the table, Aunt Marie tried to balance two toddlers on her lap because both insisted they belonged next to her. Cousin Jacob ended up in Grandpa's chair, while Grandpa stood scratching his head, muttering, "I could have sworn this was my spot."

The real mix-up came when the turkey was placed in front of Grandma. Everyone expected her to take her usual seat in the middle, but somehow she had been shuffled all the way to the head of the table. The family erupted into laughter as they realized the matriarch, who usually orchestrated everything from the sidelines, had been given the seat of honor.

"Well," Grandma said with a twinkle in her eye, "I suppose this is where I belong after all." She raised her glass, and everyone joined in a toast.

From that moment on, the confusion turned into a game. Family members swapped places between bites, pretending to take on the personalities of whoever usually sat there. Cousin Jacob imitated Grandpa's booming laugh, while Emily put on her best serious face to act like Uncle Frank.

By the end of the meal, the family decided Grandma should always sit at the head of the table. The seat swap had started as a prank, but it gave everyone a chance to laugh and remember that traditions sometimes begin by accident.

That Thanksgiving became one of the most memorable, not because of the food, but because the mix-up reminded them all that the best celebrations are filled with laughter.

The Joke That Made No Sense

Uncle Larry had a reputation for being the family comedian. At every gathering, he insisted on telling at least one of his "legendary" jokes. Some were funny, some were groan-worthy, but all were delivered with the same dramatic flair.

One summer barbecue, Larry stood up from his lawn chair, cleared his throat, and announced, "Ladies and gentlemen, prepare yourselves for the greatest joke you'll ever hear." The kids stopped tossing their football, the adults leaned in politely, and Grandma adjusted her hearing aid to make sure she caught every word.

Larry launched into a long story filled with twists, side comments, and details that seemed to go in every direction. He spoke about a farmer, a chicken, a lost shoe, and something about a train that never arrived on time. The story went on and on, and just when everyone thought it might be leading somewhere clever, Larry threw out the punchline.

Silence.

Everyone looked at one another, puzzled. The children frowned. Aunt Martha whispered to her husband, "Was that supposed to be funny?" He shrugged helplessly. Even the dog tilted its head as though waiting for an explanation.

Larry stood proudly, hands on his hips, grinning as if he had just delivered a masterpiece. When no one laughed, his grin faltered. "You didn't get it? Really?"

The pause stretched, and then cousin Ben burst into laughter—not because he understood, but because the whole moment was so awkward. His laughter set off others, until the yard was filled with giggles. Larry finally joined in, wiping his eyes. "Fine, maybe I need to work on my delivery."

From then on, the joke became a running gag. At every gathering someone would nudge Larry and say, "Tell us the chicken and train story again." He would roll his eyes, sigh dramatically, and start the tale while half the family pretended to listen with solemn faces. The punchline was always met with the same silence, followed by exaggerated applause as if he were a famous comedian finishing a set.

Larry never minded. He knew the joke itself was hopeless, but the tradition of telling it had become funnier than any punchline could ever be.

Grandma's Recipe Hiding in the Bills

In the Johnson family, Grandma Ruth's chocolate cake was legendary. Moist, rich, and topped with the perfect layer of frosting, it had been the centerpiece of every birthday and holiday for decades. So when her granddaughter Emma volunteered to bake it for the upcoming family reunion, Ruth handed her the most precious treasure: the recipe card, slightly yellowed and smudged with cocoa stains.

Emma placed the card carefully on the kitchen counter and gathered her ingredients. But when she reached for the card again, it had vanished. She checked under the flour canister, inside the cookbook, even in the trash. Nothing.

"Grandma, I think I lost it," Emma admitted nervously when Ruth called to check in.

"Lost it? That card has been in the family since 1952!" Ruth gasped.

Soon the entire household joined the search. Emma's brother emptied the utensil drawer, her father checked behind the refrigerator, and her mother flipped through every cookbook on the shelf. At one point, someone even looked in the dog's bed, just in case. The kitchen looked like a tornado had swept through.

Finally, Emma sat down at the table, defeated. She opened the stack of unpaid bills to distract herself from the disaster, and there it was: the recipe card, tucked neatly between an electric bill and a grocery coupon. She held it up triumphantly. "Found it!"

Relief turned into laughter as the family gathered around. "Of course Grandma's cake recipe would hide with the bills," her father joked. "It knows it's priceless."

Emma got to work immediately, though the chaos of the search left her a bit flustered. She misread the instructions and added too much flour, creating a cake that was taller, denser, and a little lopsided. When she presented it at the reunion, she apologized, but Grandma Ruth took a big bite and grinned.

"It may not be perfect," she said, "but it's made with love, and that's what makes it taste right."

The family agreed, enjoying every crumb of the slightly heavy cake. From that day on, the story of the lost recipe card was told alongside the serving of Grandma's cake, proof that even a mishap could turn into a memory as sweet as dessert.

A Cat at the Dinner Table

The Parker family sat down for their usual Sunday dinner, the table filled with roast chicken, mashed potatoes, and green beans. Just as everyone was serving themselves, a soft creak came from the kitchen door. At first, they thought it was the wind, but then a small gray cat strolled confidently into the dining room.

It was not their cat.

The uninvited guest leapt gracefully onto an empty chair and looked around as if to say, "I'll take my plate now." The children gasped, and Mr. Parker blinked in surprise. "Whose cat is this?" he asked.

No one answered. The cat meowed loudly, clearly unimpressed with the lack of service. Mrs. Parker, always quick to act, placed a meatball on a small plate and set it on the floor. The cat sniffed it, purred in approval, and began to eat as though it had been invited all along.

The children burst into laughter. "Can we keep him?" Emma pleaded.

"I'm not sure he belongs to us," Mrs. Parker said, though she smiled as the cat rubbed against her leg.

The rest of the dinner carried on with the cat happily munching beside them. Whenever someone dropped a crumb, the guest pounced immediately, earning cheers from the children. Mr. Parker shook his head, chuckling. "I suppose every family dinner needs a little entertainment."

After dessert, the cat calmly padded to the couch, curled into a ball, and dozed off while the Parkers cleared the table. Later, a knock came at the door. Their neighbor, Mrs. Dalton, stood outside holding a leash. "Have you seen Whiskers? He tends to wander."

The Parkers burst out laughing. "We've just had dinner with him," Mrs. Parker explained.

Mrs. Dalton apologized, but the family assured her it had been the highlight of their evening. The children waved goodbye to Whiskers as he was carried home, already asking if he could come back the next Sunday.

From then on, Whiskers made regular appearances at the Parker dinner table. Sometimes he arrived before the food, other times just in time for dessert. He was no longer a surprise guest but an honorary member of the family dinners, always guaranteed a meatball of his own.

Grandpa, the Generous Tooth Fairy

It was a big night for little Oliver. He had finally lost his first tooth and placed it carefully under his pillow, his eyes shining with excitement. "The Tooth Fairy is coming," he whispered before drifting off to sleep.

Grandpa Jack was staying over that evening, enjoying his role as the bedtime storyteller. Later that night, when everyone was asleep, he decided to help with the tradition. Still half awake, he tiptoed into Oliver's room with his wallet in hand.

The plan was simple: take the tiny tooth, leave a shiny coin, and sneak out. But in his sleepy haze, Jack fumbled. Instead of the coin, he slipped a crisp twenty-dollar bill under the pillow. Then, absentmindedly, he tucked the little tooth into his wallet and shuffled back to bed.

The next morning, Oliver woke with a squeal. "Mom! Dad! Grandpa! The Tooth Fairy left me twenty dollars!" He waved the bill high above his head like a trophy.

The entire family rushed in. His parents stared in shock, and then all eyes turned to Grandpa Jack, who was pretending to sip his coffee calmly.

"Twenty dollars?" Oliver's mom asked, raising an eyebrow.

Jack cleared his throat. "Well, maybe the Tooth Fairy was feeling generous this year."

Oliver beamed. "She must think my tooth was extra special!"

The laughter that followed filled the kitchen. Grandpa finally confessed, pulling the tiny tooth out of his wallet. "Seems the Tooth Fairy got a little confused last night."

Oliver giggled and hugged him. "You're the best Tooth Fairy ever, Grandpa."

From that day on, the story of the most generous Tooth Fairy became a family legend. Oliver told his friends at school, who begged their own parents to match the magical twenty. Grandpa Jack never lived it down, and every time another child in the family lost a tooth, he was teased with cries of, "Better watch out, the generous Tooth Fairy is coming tonight!"

Even years later, when Oliver was too old to believe in fairies, he would smile whenever he remembered that morning. For him, it was never really about the money, but about the joy of knowing his grandfather had turned a small tradition into a memory they would laugh about forever.

When the Picnic Blanket Took Off

The Wilson family loved their summer picnics at the park. On a breezy Saturday afternoon, they spread out a large checkered blanket under a shady oak tree. Baskets were unpacked, sandwiches were arranged, and lemonade was poured into plastic cups. Everything seemed perfect.

Then the wind picked up.

At first it was just a gentle flutter at the edges of the blanket. Aunt Claire placed the napkin holder on one corner, and Uncle Sam set the basket on another. But as the gusts grew stronger, the blanket began to ripple like a restless ocean.

"Hold it down!" someone shouted, but it was too late. With one mighty sweep, the wind lifted the blanket into the air, sending sandwiches tumbling and cups rolling across the grass. The family leapt up in unison, chasing after their runaway tablecloth.

Children darted through the park, laughing and shrieking, while the adults jogged awkwardly behind, trying not to spill what food was left. The blanket soared like a kite, twisting and flipping as if it had a mind of its own.

Little Ben managed to grab one corner, only to be pulled along until he collapsed in a fit of giggles. His sister Emma tried to stomp on another corner but slipped, landing softly on the grass. Even the dog joined the chase, barking joyfully as though it were all a new game.

Finally, the blanket came to rest against a row of bushes, clinging like a flag of surrender. The family gathered around, breathless and laughing, holding their rumpled picnic prize. The food was scattered, the drinks were half empty, and everyone had grass stains on their knees.

Uncle Sam dusted himself off and said, "Well, I guess the wind just wanted a bite too."

Instead of being upset, the family laid the blanket back down, this time with rocks anchoring every corner. The sandwiches were a little squished, and the cookies had crumbs everywhere, but somehow the food tasted even better after all the excitement.

As the sun dipped lower, the Wilsons agreed it was their most memorable picnic yet. The runaway blanket had turned an ordinary afternoon into a story they would tell again and again, each time with a little more laughter.

Breakfast with the Smoke Alarm

Every morning, Mr. Harris liked to make breakfast for his family. It was his way of showing love, even if cooking had never been his strength. His specialty was toast, though the results were usually questionable.

One morning, he popped four slices of bread into the toaster and hummed cheerfully as he set the table. Minutes later, the smoke alarm erupted with a loud *beep, beep, beep.*

His wife hurried in, laughing. "Not again, Harold!"

The children, already used to the routine, grabbed napkins and held them over their noses like theater masks. "Breakfast performance!" they shouted, pretending they had tickets to watch.

Mr. Harris opened the toaster to reveal four slices nearly black. "Perfectly golden," he declared, scraping them with a butter knife until crumbs scattered everywhere.

"Golden?" his daughter giggled. "Dad, they look like charcoal."

Undeterred, he placed the toast proudly on the table. The alarm still wailed until his son fanned the ceiling with a dish towel, finally silencing it.

Everyone spread jam thickly to disguise the taste. Between bites, the kids began rating each slice like judges on a cooking show. "This one's a nine for crunch," one announced. "And this one is ideal if you want extra smoke flavor," another added.

Mr. Harris bowed with a grin. "Thank you, thank you. I'll be here all week."

From then on, the family jokingly called it *The Burnt Toast Alarm Show*. Whenever the alarm sounded, they rushed to the kitchen not in panic but in anticipation of Dad's morning performance.

The toast was rarely edible, but the laughter it brought made breakfast unforgettable.

Soda Pop Shower

It was a warm summer afternoon, and the Miller family gathered in the backyard for a barbecue. The grill smoked, the potato salad was ready, and everyone was waiting for a cold drink.

Uncle Ethan brought out a two-liter bottle of soda, beads of condensation shining in the sun. "Who's ready for something fizzy?" he asked, twisting the cap with a grin.

What he didn't realize was that the bottle had been shaken during the car ride, then rolled around on the porch by the kids. The moment the cap loosened, a fountain of foam shot into the air. Soda sprayed across the table, soaking the buns, splattering the potato salad, and drenching Aunt Judy's blouse.

For a second, everyone stared in shock. Then the yard filled with laughter. "Looks like the barbecue comes with its own soda fountain," Grandpa joked, wiping his glasses.

The kids squealed with delight, darting through the spray as if it were a carnival game. Ethan stood holding the fizzing bottle, sheepish but grinning. "At least nobody's thirsty now," he said.

The family quickly cleaned up and replaced what food they could. Instead of spoiling the meal, the mishap became the day's highlight. Soon the story was being exaggerated for fun. Aunt Judy claimed the fountain had shot higher than the house, while Grandpa swore it nearly blew his hat across the yard.

By dessert, Ethan had been given a new nickname: Soda Man. At every picnic afterward, the children begged him to open the bottles, chanting, "Do it again!" The adults came prepared with paper towels, half hoping for another performance. That afternoon, sticky as it was, became one of the family's favorite memories. The exploding soda bottle proved that sometimes the best stories come not from what goes right, but from the moments that go hilariously wrong.

Too Hot to Handle Soup

Grandma Helen's chicken soup was a family treasure. Every Sunday she served it piping hot, and everyone gathered eagerly around the table. But one chilly afternoon, the soup seemed determined to stay hotter than ever.

As soon as the bowls were filled, steam poured upward in thick clouds. The family blew gently, then harder, cheeks puffed like balloons. Still, the broth was scorching.

"This soup could melt steel," joked Uncle Dave after a quick sip.

Little Lucy stirred hers furiously, while Aunt Clara tried setting her bowl near the open window. Grandpa fanned his with a napkin, muttering that they might need a fire extinguisher.

Soon the room was filled with the sound of exaggerated blowing. It was like an orchestra of brass instruments, each family member puffing away. Between bursts of laughter, they kept trying, but the soup refused to cool.

Finally, Grandma laughed and clapped her hands. "Enough of this! Let's have cookies while we wait." She brought out a tray of biscuits, and everyone nibbled happily, dipping them quickly into the broth despite the heat.

By the time the last cookie was gone, the soup had finally reached the right temperature. The first spoonfuls were delicious, perhaps even better after all the waiting and laughter.

That evening, the story became an instant favorite. Grandpa told the neighbors about their "family brass band," and the children spent days mimicking the dramatic blowing.

From then on, whenever Grandma placed soup on the table, someone always asked, "Do we need the orchestra again?" And before anyone tasted a drop, the whole room was already laughing.

Coffee Everywhere but the Cup

Every Sunday morning, Robert insisted on serving coffee to his family. He liked the little ritual of carrying steaming mugs from the kitchen to the living room, proud of being the host. The problem was that Robert always believed he could carry more than he realistically could.

One Sunday, he stacked four full cups onto a small tray. "No need to make two trips," he declared confidently, ignoring his wife's warning look. Carefully, he lifted the tray and began his slow march toward the living room.

At first, things went well. But halfway there, the cat darted across his path. Robert swerved, the tray tilted, and disaster struck.

Hot coffee splashed across the rug, the table, and, most tragically, the cat, who leapt into the air with a startled yowl. Now dripping with brown liquid, the feline dashed around the room like a wild streak, leaving spots of coffee on the sofa and curtains.

The family jumped to their feet. "Catch him!" shouted one of the kids, though no one was fast enough. By the time the cat finally dove under the couch, the living room looked like a storm had passed through.

Robert stood in the middle of the chaos, holding a tray with one lonely, half–full cup still upright. His wife put her hands on her hips, trying not to laugh. "I told you to make two trips."

The children burst out laughing, pointing at the cat now peeking out with fur sticking up in clumps. "Look, it's a cappuccino cat!" one of them shouted, and the name stuck. Cleaning up took nearly an hour, but no one was upset. Instead, the morning turned into a comedy show, complete with giggles every time the cat shook itself, sending another spray of coffee droplets into the air.

From that day on, Robert was no longer allowed to carry more than two mugs at once. And every time someone ordered a cappuccino at a café, the children would grin and whisper, "Just like our cat."

Grandpa, the Cookie Thief

Grandma's kitchen smelled heavenly on baking days. One Saturday she pulled a tray of chocolate chip cookies from the oven, golden and gooey, and set them on the counter to cool. The children crowded around, but she wagged her finger. "Not until after dinner."

When dinner was finally over, the family hurried into the kitchen. To their shock, half the cookies were gone.

"Who stole them?" Anna gasped.

The children swore they were innocent. The adults denied it too. Yet crumbs on the armchair and a wrapper peeking from under a newspaper told another story.

"The thief is clever," Uncle Ben said in his best detective voice. "But who could it be?"

The family launched a playful investigation. They checked behind curtains, under the table, even inside the breadbox. Just when it seemed the culprit would escape justice, Grandpa strolled in, whistling, with a chocolate smudge on his chin.

"Grandpa!" the kids shouted.

He froze for a moment, then grinned and pulled a half-eaten cookie from his pocket. "All right, you caught me. They were simply irresistible."

The children pounced, declaring him the most notorious bandit in the family. Instead of protesting, Grandpa leaned into the role, sneaking behind chairs and pretending to escape while the kids chased him through the living room, squealing with laughter.

When everyone collapsed on the sofa, Grandma shook her head. "The Cookie Thief strikes again."

From that night on, the children set up "cookie patrols" to guard every fresh tray. Grandpa always tried to outsmart them, sometimes winning, sometimes getting caught, but always leaving the house filled with giggles.

Spaghetti Stuck Together

Sunday dinners at the Romano household were famous for one thing: pasta. Big bowls of spaghetti, rich tomato sauce, and plenty of laughter around the table. Everyone looked forward to it, especially when Grandpa Joe was in charge of cooking.

One evening, though, Grandpa became a little too caught up in telling stories. He leaned against the counter, describing his glory days on the baseball field, while the pot of pasta bubbled furiously on the stove. The family listened, hanging on every word, completely forgetting about the timer.

By the time someone asked, "Do you smell something odd?" it was too late. Grandpa lifted the lid and groaned. Instead of perfectly cooked spaghetti, the noodles had fused into one giant, sticky mass. He poked at it with a fork, and the entire clump lifted out in a single piece, wobbling like jelly.

The family burst into laughter. "Is that pasta or modern art?" Uncle Tony teased.

Grandpa Joe, never one to lose his humor, held the mass high like a trophy. "Behold, the world's first spaghetti sculpture!"

The children clapped and cheered, delighted by the strange creation. Even Grandma, trying not to laugh, admitted it was the most memorable pasta she had ever seen.

Dinner went on with sandwiches and salad instead, but the pasta sculpture remained in the center of the table like a centerpiece. Every so often, someone poked it and giggled as the noodles wobbled.

By dessert, the story had already grown into legend. Cousin Maria claimed the spaghetti monster nearly climbed out of the pot. Uncle Tony swore he saw it blink.

From then on, whenever Grandpa cooked pasta, someone always asked, "Are we eating noodles tonight, or another sculpture?" Grandpa would wink and reply, "Depends on how good my stories are."

The Overcooked Pasta Tale became a staple of family gatherings, proving that even a kitchen disaster could turn into a feast of laughter.

A Teakettle with a Tune

In Margaret's kitchen, the old teakettle had been a loyal companion for years. Its metal was slightly dented, its handle a bit loose, but it always whistled faithfully when the water was ready for tea. One chilly morning, however, the kettle decided to change its tune.

Margaret set it on the stove as usual and went about buttering toast. Soon, instead of the sharp whistle she expected, a strange warbling sound filled the kitchen. It rose and fell like an out–of–tune trumpet, wobbling between high notes and low rumbles.

She frowned. "What on earth is that noise?"

Her husband, Harold, peeked in. "Sounds like your kettle joined the choir."

The sound grew louder, sputtering into something that almost resembled a melody. Margaret burst out laughing. "It's singing! My kettle is actually singing."

Word spread quickly. When the grandchildren arrived later that day, they begged her to make tea just so they could hear it. The moment the kettle heated up, the strange serenade began. The kids clapped in rhythm while Harold pretended to conduct an orchestra with a spoon.

The family soon gave the kettle a name: Maestro. Every time guests came over, Margaret would set it proudly on the stove and say, "Wait until you hear the show." Neighbors dropped by just to listen, leaving the kitchen in stitches as Maestro launched into another squeaky performance.

Even though the tune was far from beautiful, it became a source of endless joy. Margaret refused to replace it, insisting no fancy electric kettle could ever compete with one that sang its heart out.

One evening, Harold raised his teacup in a toast. "Here's to Maestro, the only musician in the family who never forgets his part."

The table erupted in laughter, and the kettle squealed right on cue as if agreeing.

From then on, the singing teakettle was more than just a kitchen tool. It was a reminder that sometimes the quirkiest things bring the biggest smiles.

When Sugar Tasted Salty

Baking day at Aunt Clara's house was always full of laughter. She loved inviting her nieces and nephews to help measure flour, crack eggs, and stir bowls of batter. On this particular Saturday, she promised a chocolate cake for dessert, and the children eagerly gathered in the kitchen.

Clara set out the ingredients neatly on the counter. "Now remember," she said with a wink, "baking is about following directions." The kids nodded solemnly, though their eyes sparkled with mischief.

Everything went smoothly at first. The flour puffed into the air, covering everyone in a light dusting. Eggs were cracked with only minor shell disasters. Soon the batter was glossy and rich. The last step was simple: add one cup of sugar.

Clara reached for the jar, scooped generously, and poured it into the bowl, humming happily as she stirred.

Hours later, the family gathered around the table as the cake was sliced and served. It looked perfect, with a moist crumb and smooth frosting. Everyone took a bite at the same time.

The reaction was immediate. Faces puckered, eyebrows shot up, and a chorus of coughs and groans filled the dining room.

"This cake tastes like the ocean!" one child exclaimed.

Clara rushed back to the kitchen, lifted the jar, and gasped. Instead of sugar, she had used salt. Nearly a full cup of it. She covered her face, but the family roared with laughter.

The children dared each other to take tiny bites, reacting with dramatic shudders and wild expressions. Uncle Paul even declared, "I'll finish my slice if someone brings me a pretzel to go with it."

Rather than toss it out, Clara cut the cake into small squares and placed them on a tray. The family paraded the pieces around like party favors, handing them out as a joke and awarding "prizes" to anyone brave enough to take a second bite.

By the end of the evening, the salty cake had become the entertainment. Clara promised to triple-check labels next time, but the children begged her not to. "It's the best party trick you've ever made," they teased.

From then on, whenever dessert appeared on the table, someone would whisper, "Sweet or salty?" and the whole room would laugh before anyone touched a fork.

Catch That Shopping Cart!

Saturday mornings at the supermarket were always busy, and Mr. Thompson liked to finish his shopping early. He loaded his cart with bread, fruit, and a big bag of flour, humming softly as he pushed it toward the parking lot.

The lot sloped gently downward, and Mr. Thompson paused to adjust his shopping bags. That was when it happened. He let go of the handle for just a moment, and the cart began to roll. Slowly at first, then faster, as if it had a mind of its own.

"Stop!" he shouted, chasing after it.

The cart gathered speed, rattling over bumps and clattering noisily. A woman carrying groceries stepped aside quickly, laughing as the runaway cart barreled past her. Mr. Thompson pumped his arms, trying to catch up, but the cart seemed determined to escape.

It zigzagged between parked cars, narrowly missing a bumper. The bag of flour bounced, threatening to spill. Shoppers stopped to watch, some cheering as though it were a race. One man even called out, "Run, old timer, you've got this!"

Mr. Thompson finally lunged forward, grabbing the handle just as the cart smacked gently into a row of bushes. The sudden stop sent an apple flying out, rolling across the pavement. Breathless, he bent down to retrieve it, his face flushed but grinning.

The small crowd that had gathered clapped and laughed. "Nice catch," someone said. "Almost like a game show."

Straightening his back, Mr. Thompson gave a little bow. "Thank you, thank you. I'll be signing autographs after I put away my groceries."

The audience chuckled as people drifted back to their cars. He inspected the cart. Nothing broken, and only a few squished bananas. Not too bad, considering.

When he finally got home, he told the story to his wife, who shook her head in amusement. "You went shopping and came back with exercise and applause. Not a bad trade."

From that day on, the runaway grocery cart became one of Mr. Thompson's favorite stories to tell. And each time he wheeled a cart across a parking lot, he kept a firm grip, though he secretly hoped it might try to escape again, just for the laugh.

The Day the Pie Deflated

Baking day at the Carter house was always an event. Grandma Lucy loved making pies, and everyone looked forward to her apple pie with its golden crust and sweet cinnamon filling. On one autumn afternoon, she decided to surprise the family with her masterpiece.

She worked carefully, rolling the dough until it was perfectly thin, layering the apples, and sprinkling just the right amount of sugar and spice. When the pie came out of the oven, it looked flawless. The crust was golden brown, the edges crimped neatly, and the filling bubbled gently beneath the surface.

"Isn't it beautiful?" she said proudly, setting it on the table to cool. The family gathered around, admiring it as though it were a work of art.

Finally, the moment came. Grandma sliced the pie, and everyone waited eagerly. But as soon as she lifted the first piece, the entire dessert gave a soft sigh and collapsed inward. The crust sank, the apples slid forward, and the carefully shaped masterpiece turned into a sweet, gooey puddle.

For a second, there was silence. Then Grandpa chuckled. "Looks like we're having apple soup for dessert."

The children burst into laughter, grabbing spoons instead of forks. Aunt May pretended to perform first aid, pressing napkins against the collapsed crust and shouting, "Stay with us, pie!" The living room filled with giggles as the once–perfect dessert became the star of the evening.

Despite its appearance, the pie tasted wonderful. In fact, the family declared it even better than usual. Each bite was warm, sweet, and comforting, and everyone agreed that looks were overrated when flavor was this good.

By the end of the evening, the story of the collapsing pie had already become family legend. The next time Grandma baked, the kids peeked into the oven and asked, "Is it standing strong, or ready to faint?"

Grandma laughed and replied, "Either way, it will taste delicious."

From then on, the pie that collapsed wasn't remembered as a failure but as one of the funniest and sweetest desserts the family ever shared.

Auto-Correct Strikes Again

Grandma Rose was proud of learning how to text her grandchildren. It made her feel connected and modern, even if her fingers sometimes moved slower than the tiny keys on her phone. Most of the time, her messages were short and sweet: "Love you," or "Call me soon." But one evening, auto-correct decided to play a trick on her.

She wanted to send her grandson Daniel a quick note: "Good luck on your test tomorrow. I'm proud of you." She typed carefully and pressed send. A few minutes later, her phone buzzed with Daniel's reply: a long string of laughing emojis.

Confused, Rose opened her sent messages. Instead of her thoughtful encouragement, the phone had changed her words to read: "Good duck on your toast tomorrow. I'm pruned of you."

Rose gasped, then laughed until tears filled her eyes. She quickly typed back, "Oh dear, I meant GOOD LUCK, not good duck!" but Daniel only sent more laughing faces.

Soon the whole family group chat was alive with comments. One cousin wrote, "Grandma, I'll be sure to eat toast with duck tomorrow." Another added, "Proud or pruned, either way we love you."

Rather than being embarrassed, Rose decided to embrace it. The next morning, she texted the family again: "Good duck, everyone! Stay pruned!" The responses came instantly, filled with laughter and heart emojis.

From that day on, her grandchildren crowned her the "Queen of Funny Texts." Every time her phone autocorrected a word into something silly, she saved it and shared it proudly at family dinners.

Daniel later admitted that the silly mistake had eased his nerves before the exam. "I couldn't stop laughing," he told her. "By the time I sat down for the test, I was totally relaxed. Best good-luck message ever."

Rose beamed. "Then maybe my phone knew what it was doing."

What began as a simple error became one of the family's favorite running jokes. Even years later, whenever someone had an important event, they would say, "Send us a good duck, Grandma!" And she always did, happily keeping the tradition alive.

Frozen Face on Video Chat

When the pandemic kept the family apart, weekly video calls became the new tradition. Grandpa Henry, though not very tech-savvy, was always eager to join. He loved seeing the grandchildren's faces and hearing their updates, even if connecting sometimes took a few false starts.

One Sunday afternoon, everyone logged on as usual. Faces popped up on the screen: cousins waving, parents chatting, kids showing off drawings and toys. Then Henry appeared, smiling broadly. But within seconds, his image froze.

At first, it looked normal enough. His head was tilted slightly, eyes half closed, mouth stretched into an awkward grin. The family waited, thinking the connection would clear. Instead, the frozen picture stayed.

"Grandpa?" someone called. "Can you hear us?"

His voice came through, perfectly clear. "Of course I can. Why is everyone laughing?"

The children collapsed in giggles, pointing at the screen. "Grandpa, you look like an emoji!" one shouted.

Henry tried to adjust the computer. He tapped keys, tilted the camera, and even gave the monitor a firm pat. But his frozen face remained, grinning lopsidedly at everyone. The more he moved and spoke, the funnier it became, because his still image never changed.

The cousins began taking screenshots. Within minutes, the frozen grin had been turned into stickers, funny memes, and even a birthday card design.

When Henry finally managed to unfreeze, he was met with a gallery of laughing faces. "What did I miss?" he asked innocently.

His daughter explained, showing him the screenshots. Instead of being embarrassed, Henry roared with laughter. "Well," he said, "if I can't be the smartest guy on the call, I'll settle for being the funniest."

From then on, his family nicknamed him "Grandpa Emoji." Every week, someone would tease, "Ready for your freeze face, Grandpa?" And sure enough, the joke never failed to return, sometimes by accident and sometimes on purpose when Henry leaned in and made silly faces at the camera.

What began as a technical glitch turned into one of the family's happiest traditions, reminding them that even distance could not stop the laughter.

Searching for the Wi-Fi Code

The Johnson family loved gathering at Grandma and Grandpa's house, but there was always one challenge: connecting to the Wi-Fi. No one could ever remember the password, and the paper it was written on had long since disappeared.

One Saturday afternoon, the grandchildren arrived with their phones and tablets. "Grandma, what's the Wi-Fi password?" they asked in unison.

Grandma frowned thoughtfully. "It's written down somewhere. Check the desk drawer."

The drawer revealed a jumble of old receipts, expired coupons, and a half-used book of stamps, but no password. Grandpa suggested looking in the kitchen. "I'm sure I stuck it to the fridge with a magnet," he said confidently. But the only notes on the fridge were a grocery list and a faded postcard from Florida.

The hunt grew more desperate. The kids searched under couch cushions, flipped through cookbooks, even checked the inside of the phone book. One cousin insisted it might be taped to the back of the router, but crawling behind the heavy cabinet produced only a dust bunny the size of a small cat.

Meanwhile, Grandpa settled into his chair with a newspaper. "Back in my day, we didn't need Wi-Fi," he said with a grin. The kids groaned, not in the mood for nostalgia.

After nearly an hour, frustration gave way to laughter. The whole family joined the hunt, treating it like a scavenger game. Just as they were about to give up, little Sophie shouted from the kitchen, "I found it!"

Everyone rushed over. On the side of the refrigerator, stuck under a magnet shaped like a smiling cow, was a faded note: "Wi-Fi password: GRANDKIDSWELCOME."

The kids cheered and quickly connected their devices. Grandma laughed so hard she had to sit down, while Grandpa shook his head in amusement.

Then Sophie frowned. "Wait... what's the password for Netflix?" she asked.

The room went silent for a beat before bursting into laughter again. Apparently, the next scavenger hunt had just begun.

The Lost with the GPS

Margaret and Harold loved taking weekend drives through the countryside. With a picnic basket in the backseat and the windows rolled down, it was their favorite way to spend a sunny afternoon. Margaret was in charge of navigation, but recently their children had convinced them to try using a GPS.

"Just type in the address, and it will tell you where to go," their son had explained patiently. Margaret was intrigued, while Harold was skeptical.

On their first outing with the new device, the cheerful voice instructed, "Turn right in 500 feet." Harold nodded, but when the moment came, he confidently turned left.

"Harold!" Margaret exclaimed. "It said right."

"I know where I'm going," Harold replied, gripping the wheel. The GPS paused for a moment, then calmly said, "Recalculating."

A few minutes later, the voice announced again, "Turn right at the next intersection." Harold sighed and turned left once more. Margaret buried her face in her hands, half laughing, half exasperated.

The GPS, undeterred, repeated its directions with unwavering patience. "Turn right." Harold muttered back, "You don't need to shout. I heard you the first time."

Margaret burst out laughing. "You're arguing with a machine!"

"I'm not arguing," Harold grumbled. "I'm just teaching it who's boss."

After several wrong turns and a long scenic detour, they finally arrived at the picnic spot. The basket was unpacked, the blanket spread, and the two of them sat under a tree laughing about their adventure.

"That GPS has more patience than I do," Margaret admitted.

"And worse judgment than me," Harold countered, raising his sandwich.

From that day on, the talking GPS became part of their routine. Sometimes Harold followed its directions, and sometimes he ignored them just to hear it recalculate. The grandchildren loved riding along, giggling every time Grandpa muttered back at the device.

The little machine never got upset, and Harold secretly admired its persistence. In the end, the GPS became less of a navigator and more of a travel companion, one that made every drive a little funnier.

Oops, Wrong Inbox

Grandpa William had recently discovered the joy of email. He loved sending notes to his sister in another state and enjoyed how fast it was compared to writing letters. The only trouble was that he sometimes mixed up the addresses.

One quiet afternoon, he sat at the computer and typed a long message to his sister. He wrote about his vegetable garden, the rabbits nibbling on his lettuce, and the apple pie recipe that had turned out surprisingly well. At the end, he even included a funny story about his lawn mower breaking down in the middle of the yard. Pleased with his work, he clicked send.

Later that evening, he opened his inbox and found a reply. Expecting his sister, he began to read. To his shock, the email was from his bank manager.

"Dear Mr. William," it began, "I appreciate your enthusiasm for gardening and cooking, though I believe this message was not intended for me. I especially enjoyed the pie recipe. Best regards, Mr. Collins."

Grandpa's eyes widened. He had sent his family update to the bank instead of his sister. Embarrassed, he called Margaret into the room. "Look at this. I just told our banker all about the rabbits and my apple pie!"

Margaret laughed so hard she had to sit down. "Well, at least he knows you're resourceful."

The next day, William sent a proper apology, promising to double-check addresses. To his surprise, the banker wrote back: "No worries. I've already shared your recipe with my wife, and she insists we try it this weekend."

When the family heard, they teased him endlessly. The grandchildren started calling him "Grandpa Spam," while his daughter joked that the bank might soon open a "pie account."

William laughed along, secretly pleased. His emails might have gone to the wrong inbox, but now his apple pie was famous in more than one household.

Selfie Stick Shenanigans

Nora had always been curious about new gadgets, even if they seemed a little silly. So when her granddaughter gave her a selfie stick for her birthday, she was determined to master it. "All the young people use these," Nora declared proudly. "If they can do it, so can I."

The next Sunday, the whole family gathered in the living room for a group photo. Nora extended the shiny new stick, clipped her phone in place, and held it out at arm's length. "Smile, everyone!" she said, pressing the button with confidence.

Click.

She looked at the screen. Instead of a happy family portrait, there was a clear picture of the ceiling fan.

"Well," Nora said, adjusting her glasses, "at least the fan looks cheerful."

She tried again. This time she aimed lower, but when she pressed the button, the photo captured only the tops of everyone's heads and the curtains behind them. The children giggled while her husband chuckled, "Looks like the curtains are having a family reunion."

Determined not to be defeated, Nora fiddled with the angle, muttering about technology. She stretched the stick higher, lower, sideways, even accidentally bonking Uncle Joe on the shoulder. When the next photo appeared, it showed only her own chin, magnified and glowing.

The room erupted with laughter. "Grandma, you invented modern art!" one of the kids shouted.

Finally, her granddaughter stepped in. "Here, Grandma, let me show you." She guided Nora's hand, adjusted the phone properly, and helped her press the button. At last, the screen displayed a perfect shot: smiling faces, arms wrapped around one another, and Nora beaming proudly in the center.

The family applauded, and Nora bowed dramatically. "Thank you, thank you. I am now an expert photographer."

Later, when everyone left, Nora secretly printed the ceiling fan photo and taped it to the fridge. "Just to remember where it all started," she explained with a wink.

From then on, every family gathering included Nora's selfie stick. The pictures were not always perfect, but they were always filled with laughter, and that was the kind of memory she wanted most.

Roomba vs. the Cat

When the kids bought Grandma Alice a robot vacuum, they promised it would make her life easier. "Just push a button and it cleans the whole house," her grandson explained. Alice was skeptical, but she gave it a try.

On its very first run, the little round machine zipped out of its dock with surprising speed. It hummed happily across the living room floor, bumping gently into chairs before turning and scooting in another direction. Alice followed behind with her hands on her hips. "Well, it certainly has energy," she admitted.

Then the cat noticed.

Whiskers, usually calm and dignified, arched his back and hissed as the vacuum rolled toward him. The machine paused for a second, beeped, and then continued straight ahead. Whiskers leapt into the air and bolted across the room, the vacuum rolling after him like a determined pursuer.

Alice gasped, then started laughing so hard she had to hold her side. "It's chasing the poor cat!"

The chase continued through the hallway and into the kitchen. Whiskers skidded across the tile, the robot in hot pursuit. The grandchildren, hearing the commotion, grabbed their phones and started recording. "Go, Whiskers, go!" they shouted.

At one point, the cat darted behind the sofa, only to have the robot follow and wedge itself halfway underneath. Its little wheels spun furiously, beeping as if frustrated. Whiskers perched safely on top of the armchair, glaring down like a king who had outsmarted his rival.

Finally, the battery ran low, and the vacuum gave up, returning to its dock with a pitiful beep. Whiskers flicked his tail and strutted away, victorious.

The family could not stop laughing. The video was replayed over and over, and soon it was sent to cousins, friends, and even the neighbors. Grandma Alice shook her head, still chuckling. "I thought it was supposed to clean the floors, not provide entertainment."

From then on, the vacuum was turned on only when Whiskers was outside, though the grandchildren begged to recreate the chase whenever they visited. The little machine had not only tidied up the house but also created one of the funniest family memories Alice could remember.

The Package That Wasn't Right

Mildred had recently discovered the joys of online shopping. With just a few clicks, she could order anything from books to gardening gloves without leaving her armchair. Her grandchildren encouraged her, showing her how easy it was to browse and check out.

One afternoon, she decided to treat herself to a new teapot. She searched carefully, comparing styles and colors, until she found the perfect one: a simple porcelain teapot with blue flowers painted around the edge. Pleased with her choice, she placed the order and waited eagerly for delivery.

A week later, a delivery truck pulled up. The driver struggled up the walkway with a massive cardboard box. "One package for Mildred," he said, setting it down with a thud.

Mildred blinked in confusion. "That can't be right. I only ordered a teapot."

With scissors in hand, she sliced open the box. Instead of delicate porcelain, she found a brand-new outdoor barbecue grill, shiny and enormous, complete with a bag of charcoal.

She burst out laughing, calling her daughter right away. "You'll never believe this," she said between giggles. "I ordered a teapot and ended up with a grill big enough to cook for the whole neighborhood."

That evening, the family gathered to see the mix-up. The grandchildren thought it was the funniest thing they had ever seen. "Grandma, maybe the computer thinks you're planning a party," one of them teased.

Rather than sending it back immediately, Mildred decided to embrace the surprise. "Why waste a perfectly good grill?" she said. The following weekend, she invited the neighbors over for an impromptu cookout. Burgers, hot dogs, and laughter filled the yard.

The mistaken order turned into the highlight of the summer. Every time someone asked about the new grill, Mildred grinned and replied, "Oh, that? I meant to order a teapot."

Eventually, the correct teapot arrived in a much smaller box, but by then the grill had earned a permanent place on the patio. What began as a shopping error became a source of joy, proof that sometimes the best surprises are the ones you never planned for.

The Alarm Clock That Didn't Stop

Harold had owned the same digital alarm clock for nearly twenty years. It was scratched, slightly crooked, and missing one of its rubber feet, but it had always done its job. That is, until one unforgettable Saturday morning.

At exactly seven o'clock, the clock blared its usual shrill beeping. Harold groaned, reached over, and hit the snooze button. To his surprise, the sound continued. He pressed it again, harder this time. Still the beeping went on, steady and relentless.

"Turn it off already," his wife muttered from under the covers.

"I'm trying!" Harold insisted, pressing every button he could find. He even unplugged the cord from the wall. The display went dark, but the beeping refused to stop.

Now fully awake, the family gathered in the bedroom doorway, watching as Harold wrestled with the stubborn clock. His daughter suggested taking out the batteries. He flipped it over, only to find there were no batteries at all.

"How is it still alive?" Harold shouted over the piercing noise.

They tried everything. Wrapping it in towels, burying it under cushions, even stuffing it inside a shoebox. Nothing worked. The muffled beep just kept going.

Finally, in desperation, Harold carried the buzzing device out to the backyard and dropped it in the trash bin with a triumphant slam. For a moment there was silence. Everyone held their breath. Then, faint but unmistakable, the beeping started up again from inside the can.

The family burst out laughing, clutching their sides. Harold threw up his hands. "Fine! You win!"

From then on, the alarm clock was left outside in the shed, still ticking faintly like some forgotten monster. Whenever the grandchildren visited, they would dare each other to go listen for "the ghost beep," giggling as they pressed their ears to the shed door.

Harold eventually bought a new alarm clock, but everyone agreed it never had the same personality as the one that refused to quit.

Alexa, What Did You Just Do?

When Clara's grandchildren gifted her a voice assistant for Christmas, she was delighted. The sleek little device promised to play music, give weather updates, and even tell jokes. Clara placed it proudly on the kitchen counter and immediately began experimenting.

"Play Frank Sinatra," she said clearly. The device obeyed, filling the room with music. Clara clapped her hands, thrilled.

The next day, she invited her friend Martha over for tea. "Watch this," Clara said with a grin. "It's like having a little helper." She leaned toward the device. "Turn on the radio."

Instead of music, the vacuum cleaner in the corner roared to life. Clara jumped, nearly spilling her tea, while Martha burst out laughing. "Your helper has a strange sense of humor," she said.

Clara tried again. "Stop! I said radio, not vacuum!" The machine ignored her, buzzing happily across the rug.

By then the grandchildren had gathered, laughing so hard they could hardly stand. "Grandma, you told it to connect to a device, and it chose the vacuum," one explained.

Clara threw up her hands. "So now I have a DJ that also cleans the floor?"

For the next few weeks, the mix–ups continued. When Clara asked it for the weather, it turned on the blender. When she requested a recipe, it dimmed the lights. Once, when she said "play relaxing sounds," the garage door started to open.

Despite the confusion, Clara grew fond of the little gadget. It became a source of daily entertainment. Visitors often left her house wiping tears of laughter after watching her command the assistant.

One evening, after another unexpected vacuum performance, Clara raised her teacup in a toast. "Here's to my voice assistant," she declared, "the only roommate I've ever had who argues back."

The family roared with laughter, and the device beeped as if it understood.

From then on, the assistant was less of a household tool and more of a comedy partner, reminding everyone that sometimes the best kind of technology is the kind that makes you laugh.

Sausage Thief on Four Legs

The Hendersons' backyard barbecue was in full swing. The grill sizzled, the smell of smoky sausages filled the air, and neighbors mingled with plates in hand. Everyone was laughing and enjoying the sunshine when Max, the family dog, spotted his opportunity.

Max was a friendly golden retriever with a wagging tail and a mischievous streak. He trotted around the guests, collecting pats on the head and scraps of potato chips. But his eyes were fixed on the grill, where a row of juicy sausages rested on a platter.

Grandpa set the plate on the picnic table while he went to fetch mustard. That was all Max needed. In one swift move, he leapt forward, grabbed a sausage straight off the platter, and darted across the yard with his prize dangling from his mouth.

The guests erupted in laughter. "There he goes!" shouted Uncle Pete, spilling his drink as he tried to give chase. Children squealed with delight, cheering Max on as if it were a race.

The golden retriever bounded in circles, ears flopping, sausage clenched tight. Every time someone got close, he dodged away, tail wagging furiously. Even the neighbors joined the chase, turning the barbecue into a comedy show.

Finally, Max plopped down triumphantly under the shade of a tree, licking his chops with satisfaction. The sausage was gone, and his expression made it clear he had no regrets.

Grandpa shook his head, chuckling. "Well, at least he only took one."

The family quickly replaced the missing sausage, but the story of Max's daring theft overshadowed the rest of the meal. For the rest of the afternoon, the guests teased Grandpa, saying, "Better guard your plate, or Max will strike again."

The children later drew pictures of Max the "Sausage Thief," complete with a superhero cape. Grandma pinned one to the fridge, declaring Max the official mascot of family cookouts.

From that day forward, whenever the Hendersons held a barbecue, Max was watched as closely as the grill. And every time a sausage sizzled, someone would grin and say, "Careful, the thief is on patrol."

What started as a stolen bite became one of the family's favorite memories, proving that sometimes the best part of a meal is the story that comes with it.

Yarn Basket Cat Nap

Eleanor loved to knit. Her living room was filled with colorful yarn, half–finished scarves, and a cozy basket where she kept her supplies. One rainy afternoon, she settled into her armchair, ready to spend a few quiet hours working on a blanket for her granddaughter.

But the basket was no longer empty.

Curled up inside, purring contentedly, was her cat, Daisy. The gray tabby had made herself quite comfortable among the balls of yarn, her paws tucked neatly under her chin. Eleanor sighed with a smile. "Of all the spots in this house, you had to pick this one."

When Eleanor gently reached for a ball of blue yarn, Daisy opened one eye and batted it playfully. The yarn rolled across the floor, unraveling as it went. Soon Daisy leapt after it, sending strands flying under the table and around the legs of chairs.

Within minutes, the tidy knitting corner looked like a web of colorful spaghetti. Daisy dashed through the loops, tangling herself and the furniture in a wild game. Eleanor tried to keep up, laughing as she stumbled across the room, knitting needles in hand.

By the time Daisy flopped onto her back, panting happily, the living room was a chaotic masterpiece of twisted yarn. Eleanor stood in the middle of it all, shaking her head but unable to stop laughing. "I suppose you've turned my hobby into modern art."

When her grandchildren arrived later that day, they gasped at the sight. "Grandma, did you knit a jungle?" one of them asked, eyes wide. Daisy meowed proudly as if to say, "Yes, I did."

Instead of being annoyed, Eleanor decided to leave the mess until after dinner. The children joined in, weaving the yarn into silly shapes and crowns for Daisy, who strutted around like royalty.

From that day forward, the knitting basket no longer belonged entirely to Eleanor. It became Daisy's throne, her favorite spot for napping and mischief. And whenever Eleanor picked up her needles, she always checked first to see if her little helper was already on the job.

Parrot Playing Telephone

The Simmons family had a parrot named Oliver, a bright green bird with a sharp beak and an even sharper sense of humor. He had lived with them for years, mimicking laughter, whistles, and the occasional "hello" when guests walked through the door. But no one expected the trick he pulled one rainy afternoon.

The family was gathered in the living room, sipping tea and playing cards, when the familiar sound of the telephone rang from the kitchen. Grandma hurried to answer it, but when she lifted the receiver, there was only silence.

"That's strange," she murmured, returning to her seat.

Moments later, the phone rang again. Grandpa grumbled and went to pick it up. Once more, there was no one on the line.

This continued three more times. Each time the phone rang loudly, and each time the family rushed to answer it, only to be met with silence. Finally, Grandpa threw up his hands. "Our phone is haunted."

That was when Oliver squawked from his perch, "Ring, ring! Ring, ring!"

The family froze, then burst into laughter. It had been Oliver all along, perfectly imitating the phone. He flapped his wings proudly as if bowing after a performance.

From then on, Oliver used his new trick at every opportunity. Whenever someone sat down with a book, he would interrupt with a loud "Ring, ring!" sending them rushing to the kitchen before realizing they had been fooled. Sometimes he followed up with a cheeky "Hello? Hello?" in Grandma's exact voice, which only made everyone laugh harder.

The grandchildren loved showing him off to their friends. "Watch this," they would say, and Oliver never failed to deliver his famous prank. Guests often left the Simmons house with sore cheeks from laughing so much.

What began as a moment of confusion turned into one of the parrot's most beloved routines. And while the family still jumped occasionally at the phantom phone calls, they would always smile afterward, grateful that Oliver's antics kept their home filled with laughter.

Hamster on the Loose

When little Tommy got a hamster for his birthday, he named him Houdini, certain the tiny creature was destined for great adventures. The furry escape artist did not disappoint.

One evening, while the family was watching television, Tommy peeked into the cage and gasped. "He's gone!" The door to the hamster's cage hung wide open, the bedding ruffled and empty.

The living room instantly erupted into chaos. Tommy grabbed a flashlight, his sister crawled under the couch, and their parents began moving furniture. "Check the corners," Dad said. "He can't have gone far."

But Houdini was nowhere to be found. The search continued into the kitchen, where flour had been scattered suspiciously near the pantry. "He's leaving us clues," Tommy whispered dramatically, as though they were on a treasure hunt.

For two hours, the family combed through the house. They opened cabinets, peeked into shoes, and even checked the laundry basket. Just when everyone was ready to give up, Grandma shuffled into the hallway carrying her slippers. She stopped, frowned, and lifted one slowly.

There, curled inside the warm slipper, was Houdini himself, looking quite pleased with his cozy hiding spot. His tiny nose twitched as if to say, "What took you so long?"

The family burst into relieved laughter. Tommy scooped him up gently, kissing the top of his furry head. "You really are Houdini," he said.

That night, Dad reinforced the cage door with extra clips, but the legend of Houdini the escape artist was already born. For weeks, whenever the family told the story, they exaggerated it a little more. Uncle Jim claimed the hamster had been halfway to the neighbor's yard, while Tommy insisted he saw paw prints leading toward the cookie jar.

The slipper became a family joke too. Grandma refused to wear it again, declaring it "Hamster Headquarters," and the children often placed treats inside it to see if Houdini would return.

Though the great escape had lasted only a few hours, it became one of the family's favorite tales, proving that sometimes the smallest pets create the biggest adventures.

Goldfish with a Starring Role

The Parker family thought a goldfish would be the easiest pet in the world. No barking, no scratching, no mess. Just a little swimming companion in a bowl on the kitchen counter. They named him Bubbles, certain he would spend his days quietly circling in peace.

Bubbles, however, had other plans.

Every morning, as soon as someone entered the kitchen, he would dart to the front of the glass and tap his tiny nose against it. At first, the family thought it was coincidence. But then they noticed he did it again and again, each time someone walked in.

"Look at him," said Anna, laughing. "He's saying good morning."

The habit grew stronger. Bubbles began swimming frantically in circles, splashing the surface until drops of water landed on the counter. If no one paid attention, he flicked his tail harder, making a little wave that seemed like a demand.

Soon it became impossible to ignore him. Dad joked, "I think we adopted a diva."

The children decided to test his behavior. Whenever they applauded or clapped, Bubbles swam even faster, tapping the glass as though soaking up the applause. Grandma laughed so hard she nearly dropped her spoon. "He's not a goldfish. He's a performer!"

Word spread quickly. When neighbors came over, the kids proudly introduced their star pet. "Watch this," they said, clapping their hands. True to form, Bubbles whirled around, tail flicking like a drumbeat, and tapped the glass until the visitors applauded.

The Parker kitchen soon became the stage for daily shows. Morning greetings turned into full performances, with the family cheering and Bubbles responding like the star of an aquarium circus.

One evening, as they gathered for dinner, Dad raised his glass. "Here's to Bubbles, the goldfish who refuses to be ordinary." Everyone laughed, and Bubbles swam proudly to the front of his bowl as if acknowledging the toast.

What was meant to be a simple pet became one of the family's greatest sources of joy. Bubbles wasn't just a fish in a bowl. He was a tiny performer who taught the Parkers that sometimes even the smallest creatures want a little applause.

Best Friends: Dog and Postman

Most dogs bark furiously when the mail carrier approaches. They growl, scratch at the door, and treat every delivery like a threat. But not Buddy.

Buddy was a golden Labrador with a heart as big as his wagging tail. From the day the Parkers brought him home, he seemed to adore everyone he met, but his favorite visitor of all was Mr. Jenkins, the neighborhood mail carrier.

The first time they met, Buddy bounded to the door with excitement. Instead of barking, he sat down politely, tail thumping, and waited. Mr. Jenkins laughed, bent down, and scratched Buddy behind the ears. From that moment, the friendship was sealed.

Every morning after that, Buddy would sit by the window, ears perked, watching for the familiar blue uniform. The second he spotted Mr. Jenkins, Buddy would leap up, spinning in circles until the door opened.

Mr. Jenkins soon learned to bring an extra biscuit in his pocket. "Special delivery for Buddy," he would say, slipping the treat through the crack in the door. Buddy would wag so hard his whole body shook, then follow Mr. Jenkins down the sidewalk with a look of pure devotion.

Neighbors began to notice. "Your dog's the only one who waits for the mail like it's Christmas morning," one of them joked.

The friendship grew into a daily ritual. Rain or shine, Buddy greeted the mail with joy. On snowy mornings, Mr. Jenkins would brush snow off Buddy's fur while Buddy licked his gloves. In summer, Buddy stretched out in the yard while Mr. Jenkins refilled his water bowl before continuing his route.

One day, when a substitute mail carrier arrived, Buddy sat by the door wagging expectantly. But when the stranger dropped the letters without stopping, Buddy let out a disappointed whine. That evening, Mr. Jenkins returned on his own time just to give Buddy his biscuit, laughing at the dog's delighted reaction.

Over the years, Buddy grew slower, but he never missed a morning at the window. And every day, without fail, Mr. Jenkins made sure his favorite customer received his delivery.

It became a friendship that outlasted packages and letters, a reminder that sometimes the smallest routines create the biggest bonds.

Neighborhood Watch Cat

Mrs. Turner's house sat on a quiet street where not much happened. Neighbors mowed their lawns, children rode their bikes, and cars rolled slowly by. But for years, there was one constant source of entertainment: her cat, Misty, who loved to sit in the big front window.

Every morning, as soon as the sun rose, Misty leapt onto the wide windowsill, curled her tail neatly around her paws, and began her daily watch. She wasn't content to simply lounge. No, Misty took her role very seriously, as though she were the guardian of the street.

Whenever someone walked by, Misty's ears perked up and her eyes followed them carefully. If it was a jogger, she crouched low like a hunter. If it was a dog on a leash, she tapped the glass with her paw, her whiskers twitching in indignation. Delivery trucks were met with a flick of her tail and an intense stare, as if she were inspecting their credentials.

At first, the neighbors laughed quietly to themselves, but soon Misty became a local celebrity. Children waved at her on their way to school. The mail carrier greeted her with a cheerful, "Morning, Officer Misty." Even joggers slowed down just to chuckle at the vigilant cat in the window.

Mrs. Turner, amused, began leaving little notes taped to the window. One read, "Security on Duty." Another said, "Misty is watching you." These small jokes delighted the neighbors even more.

One Halloween, the kids even dressed up as "Misty's Patrol," wearing paper badges and pretending to take orders from the cat behind the glass. Misty sat proudly in her post, blinking slowly as if approving her squad.

Over time, Misty's watch became part of the rhythm of the street. People would mention her at block parties and even include her in neighborhood newsletters. "Misty reported no suspicious activity this month," one update read.

Though she was only a housecat, Misty gave the community a reason to smile each day. For Mrs. Turner, it was heartwarming to know her beloved pet had become such a fixture in people's lives.

And so, Misty kept her post, morning after morning, reminding everyone that sometimes the smallest guardians bring the greatest comfort.

Goat in the Living Room

During a summer visit to her cousin's farm, Clara expected to enjoy fresh air, homemade pie, and maybe a ride on the tractor. What she did not expect was to meet the most troublesome goat in the county.

The goat's name was Charlie, though everyone called him Trouble. He had a knack for sneaking into places he didn't belong. Fences were no obstacle, and locked gates only seemed to encourage him. Clara first met him when he trotted boldly onto the porch, chewing on a kitchen towel he had stolen from the clothesline.

"Charlie!" Cousin Henry shouted, but the goat only flicked his ears and kept chewing.

The real chaos began when the family gathered outside for lemonade. Charlie spotted the group, lowered his head, and strutted toward them as if he were the guest of honor. Before anyone could stop him, he snatched Uncle Bill's straw hat straight off his head and pranced around the yard, showing off his new prize.

Children squealed with laughter, chasing after him. Each time someone came close, Charlie darted away, leaping onto picnic benches and knocking over cups of lemonade. At one point, he managed to grab a paper napkin in his mouth, leaving a trail of soggy shreds behind him.

Clara could not stop laughing, even as she tried to help. "He's faster than a dog!" she exclaimed.

Eventually, Cousin Henry lured Charlie back with a handful of corn. The goat trotted over innocently, dropping the crumpled hat at Uncle Bill's feet as if nothing had happened. With his mouth full of corn, he looked perfectly pleased with himself.

The family spent the rest of the afternoon swapping stories about Charlie's past adventures. Apparently, he had once climbed onto the roof of the barn and another time chased the mail carrier down the lane. "He thinks he owns the place," Henry admitted with a grin.

By the time Clara returned home, Charlie had become her favorite memory of the visit. Whenever she told the story, she described him not as a nuisance but as the farm's greatest entertainer.

And on that farm, everyone agreed: life was never dull with Charlie the mischievous goat around.

Picnic Basket Stowaway

The Wilson family loved Sunday picnics at the park. They would pack sandwiches, fruit, and a big thermos of lemonade into a wicker basket, spread a blanket under a shady tree, and spend the afternoon playing games and sharing food.

One sunny afternoon, as everyone settled down to eat, little Emma reached into the basket for an apple. Instead of fruit, her hand touched something warm and furry. She yelped and pulled back, eyes wide.

The basket gave a small wiggle, followed by a faint whimper. Curious, the family leaned in as Dad carefully lifted the lid. To everyone's astonishment, a floppy-eared puppy poked his head out, blinking in the sunlight.

The children squealed with delight. "A puppy! A real puppy!"

The little dog wriggled free, tumbling onto the blanket and scattering napkins as he rolled over and wagged his tail. He bounded from one family member to the next, showering them with licks and nibbles. Grandma laughed so hard her glasses nearly slipped off.

"Where on earth did he come from?" Mom asked, still giggling as the puppy tried to climb into the potato salad.

They looked around the park, expecting someone to come running, but no one did. The puppy seemed to have wandered over and curled up in their basket while they weren't looking.

The children immediately voted to keep him. "Please, please, can we take him home?" Emma begged, hugging the pup tightly.

Dad hesitated, but when the puppy nestled into his lap and fell asleep, even he couldn't resist. "All right," he sighed with a smile. "But only if we make sure no one's missing him."

After asking around and posting a notice at the park, it became clear the puppy had been abandoned. So the Wilsons welcomed him into their family, naming him Biscuit after the picnic where they had found him.

From that day on, Biscuit joined every outing. He learned to chase frisbees, beg for sandwiches, and nap on the blanket in the sunshine.

The story of the puppy in the picnic basket became one of the family's happiest memories, a reminder that sometimes the best surprises are the ones that wiggle their way right into your heart.

Bus-Riding Cat

In the small town of Maplewood, the morning bus always carried the same mix of commuters: office workers with coffee cups, students with backpacks, and one very unusual passenger. His name was Smokey, a sleek gray cat who rode the bus almost every day.

No one knew exactly when Smokey started his routine. Some said he first followed his owner to the stop and simply decided to hop on. Others believed he liked the warmth of the bus on chilly mornings. Whatever the reason, Smokey quickly became a regular.

At precisely eight o'clock, he trotted onto the bus with the confidence of someone who had already paid the fare. The driver, Mr. Collins, greeted him warmly. "Morning, Smokey."

The cat would leap onto an empty seat, curl his tail neatly around his paws, and watch the world go by through the window. Passengers smiled, snapping photos and shaking their heads. Smokey behaved better than most riders. He never made noise, never caused trouble, and always seemed to know when it was time to get off.

At his usual stop near the park, Smokey would hop down the aisle and wait patiently for the doors to open. He would stretch, flick his tail, and trot off as though he had important business to attend to. Sometimes children followed him, curious about where he went, only to see him lounging in the sunshine near the fountain.

The town grew fond of its four-legged commuter. The local newspaper even ran a story titled "The Cat Who Rides the Bus," complete with a photo of Smokey gazing out the window like a thoughtful traveler. Tourists passing through Maplewood often asked which bus to take just to catch a glimpse of him.

One afternoon, a passenger joked, "We should get him his own bus pass." The next week, the driver taped a little cardboard card to the window with Smokey's name on it. Everyone laughed, and Smokey seemed to approve with a slow blink.

Over time, Smokey became more than just a curiosity. He was a reminder of the town's charm, a daily surprise that made people smile before work or school.

And so, the cat who rode the bus became a local legend, proving that sometimes the best passengers are the ones who never say a word.

The Man with the Crooked Hat

Mr. Albert was known all over town for one thing: his old brown hat. It had been his faithful companion for decades, worn on fishing trips, family picnics, and countless walks through Main Street. The problem was that no matter how carefully he put it on, the hat always sat at an angle, slightly crooked to one side.

At first, people tried to help. "Albert, your hat's slipping," the barber would say, reaching up to adjust it. Within minutes, however, it tilted again, as if the hat itself preferred being lopsided.

Children giggled when they saw him coming, whispering, "There goes Mr. Crooked Hat!" Teenagers teased gently, and even the mayor once offered to buy him a new one. But Albert only smiled. "This hat has character. Why would I trade it for something ordinary?"

Over time, the crooked hat became a part of his identity. On Main Street, shopkeepers greeted him with a cheerful, "Looking sharp today, Albert," while neighbors affectionately tilted their own caps in imitation. He responded with a wink and a tip of his hat, proud of the attention.

One summer, the town held its annual parade. Albert joined the march, walking proudly in his crooked hat. The crowd clapped and laughed, and someone shouted, "Make way for our fashion icon!" The local photographer snapped a picture that ended up in the newspaper with the caption, "Main Street's Most Stylish."

From that day forward, Albert embraced his role as the town's accidental trendsetter. Young people started wearing their caps slightly tilted, calling it "the Albert look." He found the whole thing hilarious but secretly enjoyed being recognized.

Years later, when he was asked why he never straightened the hat, Albert chuckled. "Life's a little crooked sometimes, and that makes it more interesting. My hat just reminds me of that."

Main Street never forgot its beloved character. Even after Albert passed the hat down to his grandson, people still smiled when they saw it tilted to the side. The crooked hat had become a symbol of charm, laughter, and the joy of not taking oneself too seriously.

Sing-Along on the City Bus

The morning bus ride was usually quiet. Passengers scrolled through their phones, sipped coffee, or stared sleepily out the windows. That all changed one Friday when Mrs. Caldwell, carrying her grocery bags, hummed a familiar tune as she climbed aboard.

She sat down, still humming, and the sound caught the ear of a young man nearby. He smiled, recognized the melody, and softly joined in. A woman a few rows back added her voice, and before long, the whole bus was filled with the gentle strains of an old folk song.

The driver glanced in the mirror, amused. "If you're going to sing," he called out, "sing loud enough so I can hear too." That was all the encouragement they needed. The volume rose, harmonies wove together, and laughter bubbled between verses.

Some passengers clapped along, while others swayed in their seats. One little girl stood on the bench and waved her arms like a conductor. Her mother laughed, and the crowd followed her lead, singing even louder.

When the song ended, there was a moment of silence before someone started another, this time a lively tune everyone knew. The bus transformed into a rolling concert hall. Strangers who had never spoken before shared smiles and verses, their morning commute turned into a celebration.

As the bus neared downtown, the driver slowed at a red light and, to everyone's surprise, joined in himself. His deep baritone voice filled the air, earning cheers from the passengers.

When the bus finally reached its stop, no one seemed eager to leave. People lingered in the aisle, still humming, reluctant to let the moment end. Mrs. Caldwell gathered her bags and grinned. "Best bus ride I've ever had," she said.

From that day forward, the Friday sing–along became a tradition. Commuters looked forward to it all week, and the driver even kept a small stack of lyric sheets taped near his seat.

What began as one woman's humming grew into a joyful ritual that made ordinary mornings unforgettable. And every time the voices rose together, the bus became more than transportation. It became a community on wheels.

Sitting in the Wrong Row

The town theater was buzzing with excitement on Saturday night. Couples filed in, friends greeted each other in the lobby, and the ushers guided people toward their seats. Among the crowd were Henry and Martha, dressed in their best clothes and eager to enjoy the evening performance.

They found what they believed were their seats, two plush chairs in the middle row with a perfect view of the stage. Settling in, Henry removed his hat and sighed contentedly. "Perfect spot," he whispered to Martha.

Moments later, a younger couple approached, holding tickets. "Excuse us," the man said politely, "but I think you might be in our seats."

Henry frowned and checked his stub. "Row G, seats 12 and 13," he read aloud. "That's what we have."

"That's what ours say too," the woman replied, showing her ticket.

Confused, they all compared stubs again. The usher was called, and after a careful look, she smiled kindly. "You're both correct, but you're in different sections. This is Row G of the left balcony. Your seats are Row G of the right balcony."

Henry and Martha blinked at each other. "Well," Henry said with a chuckle, "no wonder these seats seemed too good to be true."

The younger couple laughed, insisting it was no trouble. The whole situation turned lighthearted as the usher guided Henry and Martha across the theater. Along the way, people in the nearby rows, curious about the confusion, began smiling and whispering.

By the time the couple finally sat in the correct seats, they were laughing so hard they could barely catch their breath. Martha wiped a tear from her eye. "At least we got a standing ovation on the way here," she said, noting the amused looks from other theatergoers.

Later, during intermission, they bumped into the younger couple in the lobby. Both pairs laughed again, swapping stories about the mix–up. "Next time," Henry joked, "we'll just follow you to the right section."

The mistake became part of the night's entertainment, and when the curtain closed at the end of the show, Henry and Martha agreed it had been one of their most enjoyable evenings. Not just because of the play, but because of the unexpected comedy of finding the wrong theater seat.

Umbrellas Dancing in the Parade

The annual spring parade was a beloved tradition in Milltown. Families lined the sidewalks, children waved flags, and vendors sold popcorn and balloons. This particular year, though, the weather had other plans. Dark clouds gathered overhead, and as the marching band turned onto Main Street, the first drops of rain began to fall.

In seconds, umbrellas popped open all along the parade route, turning the street into a sea of bright colors. Red, yellow, blue, and green domes dotted the crowd, creating a cheerful shield against the drizzle. For a while, it seemed as though the rain would not dampen the spirits of the townspeople.

Then the wind picked up.

At first it was a gentle breeze, tugging at jacket sleeves and making flags ripple. But within minutes, a powerful gust swept through the street. Dozens of umbrellas flipped inside out at the same time, their spokes bending awkwardly as fabric flapped wildly.

The sight was so sudden and so ridiculous that laughter rippled through the crowd. People struggled to wrestle their rebellious umbrellas back into shape while the band tried to keep marching in step. One tuba player nearly toppled over as his umbrella turned into a giant funnel, catching the wind like a sail.

Children squealed with delight, pointing at the colorful chaos. Some spectators gave up entirely, abandoning their umbrellas and choosing instead to dance in the rain. The entire scene looked less like a parade and more like a comedy show.

Even the performers could not resist joining in. The baton twirlers raised their soggy sticks in salute, and the drummers pounded out a playful rhythm to match the commotion. The crowd clapped along, cheering louder than before.

By the time the rain slowed and the wind eased, no one seemed to mind being wet. Umbrellas lay scattered and broken along the curb, but spirits were higher than ever. People hugged, laughed, and agreed it had been the most memorable parade in years.

Later, when photos appeared in the local paper, the headline read, *Milltown Marches On: Rain, Wind, and Laughter Steal the Show*. And every time someone mentioned the spring parade, the first image that came to mind was not the floats or the bands, but the unforgettable umbrella ballet on Main Street.

Pumpkins That Weren't for Dinner

Every Saturday morning, Mr. Daniels visited the farmer's market. He loved the colorful stalls, the smell of fresh bread, and the cheerful chatter of vendors calling out their specials. That week, he had one mission: buy pumpkins for the family's weekend dinner.

He strolled past baskets of apples and jars of honey until he reached a stand stacked with small, round pumpkins. They looked perfect, bright orange and neatly arranged. Mr. Daniels filled a bag with three of them, whistling as he paid the vendor.

Back home, his wife Clara clapped her hands. "Wonderful! We'll make pumpkin soup tonight." She began chopping onions while Mr. Daniels cut into the first pumpkin. Instead of soft, rich flesh, his knife scraped against something hard and dry. He frowned and tried again. The pumpkin crumbled oddly under the blade.

"These don't look right," he muttered.

Clara peeked over his shoulder and burst out laughing. "Oh, Harold, these aren't cooking pumpkins. They're decorative ones!"

Sure enough, the label on the bag still read "Decorative Gourds – Not Edible." Mr. Daniels had been so focused on finding something orange and round that he never bothered to read the sign.

The children crowded into the kitchen, giggling at their father's mistake. "So are we eating painted wood tonight?" one of them teased.

Clara shook her head, still laughing. "Well, we can't make soup, but we do have beautiful centerpieces for the table." She arranged the little gourds in a bowl, and suddenly the kitchen looked ready for autumn.

Not wanting to waste the moment, Mr. Daniels dashed back to the market for proper pumpkins. When he returned, the family helped prepare a delicious, hearty soup. As they ate, the decorative gourds sat proudly in the middle of the table, a reminder of his mix-up.

From then on, whenever the Daniels went shopping, someone would whisper, "Check the label, Dad," and the whole family would laugh. The decorative gourds stayed on the table all season long, not as food but as the funniest shopping mistake the family had ever enjoyed.

Melting Ice Cream Mayhem

It was the hottest day of summer, the kind of afternoon when even the trees seemed too tired to move. The Ramirez family decided the only cure was a trip to the ice cream stand at the park. With cones piled high and sprinkles scattered generously, they found a shady bench and settled down to enjoy their treats.

At first everything was perfect. The kids licked happily, Grandpa hummed with delight over his vanilla scoop, and even the dog sat patiently, hoping for a bite. But the blazing sun was merciless. Before long, streams of melted ice cream began sliding down the sides of the cones.

"Eat faster!" shouted little Sofia, as chocolate dripped onto her shirt.

Her brother Mateo tried to lick around his cone to catch every drop, but the melting outpaced him. Soon, his hands were coated in sticky strawberry, and the dog seized the opportunity, licking his fingers with glee.

Grandpa's vanilla scoop lasted the longest, but even he was not spared. One moment he was savoring a slow bite, the next his scoop slid right off the cone and landed with a soft splat on the pavement. He stared in disbelief before bursting into laughter. "Well," he said, "I guess the sidewalk was hungry too."

By now, everyone was a sticky mess. Sprinkles clung to fingers, shirts were smeared with fudge, and the dog wore a smear of strawberry across his nose. Passersby chuckled at the sight of the family, who looked more like they had lost a food fight than enjoyed dessert.

Instead of giving up, Clara, the mother, rallied the group. She marched them to the stand and ordered cups instead of cones. "Lesson learned," she said with a grin. "Ice cream is for spoons on days like this."

Back on the bench, they finished their treats neatly, though the laughter over the meltdown lasted longer than the ice cream itself.

For the rest of the summer, whenever someone suggested cones, Grandpa would wag his finger. "Careful, or you'll end up feeding the sidewalk again." And the memory of that sticky, hilarious afternoon became one of the family's sweetest stories.

The Suitcase That Refused to Follow

Travel days were always hectic for Margaret and George. Between packing snacks, remembering tickets, and keeping track of their hats, they already had their hands full. But nothing challenged them quite like George's old suitcase.

It was one of those rolling bags with a retractable handle, purchased many years earlier when George believed it would make travel "effortless." In truth, the suitcase seemed to have a will of its own.

At the train station one summer morning, George tugged it confidently behind him. At first it rolled smoothly, but as soon as the platform grew crowded, the suitcase decided to misbehave. Instead of following in a straight line, it spun sideways, colliding gently with a bench. George pulled harder, muttering under his breath. The bag swiveled again, now veering sharply toward a potted plant.

"George," Margaret called, trying not to laugh, "I think your suitcase has had too much coffee."

Determined to regain control, George straightened the handle and tried again. The suitcase wobbled like a mischievous puppy on a leash, circling his legs until he nearly tripped. Commuters smiled as they stepped aside, watching the battle between man and luggage.

By the time they reached the ticket gate, George was red-faced but grinning. "This blasted thing is testing my patience," he said, wrestling it back into line.

The final challenge came on the escalator. The suitcase refused to roll forward, as if planting its wheels in protest. George gave it a firm tug, nearly losing his balance as the bag finally lurched onto the step. Margaret clutched the railing, laughing so hard tears rolled down her cheeks.

When they finally boarded the train, the suitcase toppled onto its side with a dramatic thud. George sat down beside it, wiping his brow. "Victory," he declared, "but barely."

Throughout the ride, fellow passengers chuckled whenever they glanced at the stubborn bag. One even leaned over and whispered, "Looks like it needs its own ticket." From that day on, the suitcase was no longer just luggage. It became a family legend, remembered at every holiday and gathering. The story of George's wrestling match with his rolling suitcase reminded everyone that sometimes the journey is more entertaining than the destination.

Comedians on the Park Bench

On sunny afternoons, Mr. Lewis and his longtime friend Arthur met at the park. They always chose the same wooden bench near the fountain, a spot that gave them a clear view of people strolling by. For most visitors, it was just a seat. For Lewis and Arthur, it was a stage.

The two men had a gift for turning ordinary observations into comedy. When a jogger went past, Lewis whispered, "There goes the town's fastest delivery man, except he's forgotten the mail." Arthur followed up with, "And his shoelaces too." The pair chuckled until their shoulders shook.

A little boy dropped his ice cream cone, and Arthur leaned toward Lewis. "That's a tragedy in three acts," he said solemnly. Lewis added, "Act four will be the cleanup," as the child's mother hurried in with napkins.

Soon their laughter began attracting attention. Passersby slowed down, curious about what was so funny. A group of teenagers sat on the grass nearby, listening and giggling at the running commentary. Even the park's groundskeeper paused his work to smirk at their jokes.

One afternoon, a woman with a stroller stopped right in front of them. "You two ought to have your own show," she said. "You're funnier than the television."

Arthur tipped his hat. "The Park Bench Comedy Hour, every afternoon at three," he announced.

Word spread quickly. Regular visitors began timing their walks to coincide with the men's bench sessions. People would bring coffee, sit nearby, and wait for the improvised humor to begin. Sometimes Lewis and Arthur joked about the pigeons, calling them "the official marching band of the park." Other times, they created elaborate backstories for strangers, turning every passerby into a character.

Though nothing was scripted, the laughter was real and contagious. The bench became known as the park's unofficial comedy corner, where anyone could stop for a smile.

Years later, the park staff even placed a small plaque on the bench that read, "To Lewis and Arthur, who proved that laughter is best shared outdoors."

And so the park bench comedy show lived on, remembered not just for the jokes but for the joy it brought to everyone who passed by.

The Wrong Bus Ticket

It had been years since Helen had taken the bus. Most days she preferred walking or catching a ride with her daughter, but on that Saturday she decided to be adventurous. She bought a ticket at the station, glanced quickly at the printed slip, and boarded what she thought was the bus to the downtown market.

At first, everything seemed normal. She settled into a window seat, smiling at the people around her. The driver started the engine, and the bus rolled out of the station. Helen relaxed, imagining herself buying fresh flowers and fruit in less than half an hour.

But after twenty minutes, she noticed the scenery was unfamiliar. Instead of tall buildings and busy streets, she saw wide fields, barns, and grazing cows. Puzzled, she leaned toward the woman sitting beside her. "Excuse me, does this bus go to the market?"

The woman chuckled kindly. "Oh no, dear. This bus goes to Fairview, the little town by the lake."

Helen's eyes widened. "Fairview? I only meant to go downtown!" She checked her ticket again and laughed at her mistake. She had boarded the wrong bus entirely.

When the driver overheard, he smiled in the mirror. "Don't worry, ma'am. Fairview is a nice place. You might even enjoy it."

And he was right. By the time the bus reached the small town, Helen had made friends with two other passengers who promised to show her around. Instead of shopping at the market, she spent the day exploring a charming craft fair, sampling homemade fudge, and sitting by the lake with an ice cream cone.

When she finally returned home, her daughter asked, "So, did you get your groceries?"

Helen grinned. "No groceries. But I found a fair, a lake, and the best fudge I've ever eaten."

From then on, the family teased her every time she traveled. "Make sure you read your ticket, Mom," her daughter would say with a wink.

Helen never minded. The wrong bus ticket had given her one of the most delightful days she could remember. And whenever she passed the bus station, she smiled at the thought that sometimes the best journeys are the ones you never planned.

The Seaside Sandcastle Collapse

The Mitchell family loved spending summer weekends at the beach. They packed towels, umbrellas, and a cooler full of sandwiches, but what they enjoyed most was building sandcastles. Each year, they tried to outdo themselves, adding towers, bridges, and moats to their creations.

One bright afternoon, the children declared, "This year we'll build the biggest castle yet!" Buckets and shovels clattered as they set to work. Mom sketched out the plan in the sand, while Dad fetched buckets of water to pack the walls tightly. The grandparents joined in too, carefully shaping little windows with seashells.

Hours passed, and the castle grew taller and more impressive. There were turrets with seashell flags, winding stairways, and even a moat filled with seawater. Beachgoers stopped to admire the masterpiece. Some took pictures, while others offered compliments. "Looks like something out of a fairy tale," one woman said.

At last, the family stood back to admire their work. "Perfect," Dad said proudly. "This one might last until tomorrow."

But the ocean had other ideas.

A strong wave rolled closer, then another, each creeping nearer to the carefully dug moat. The children tried frantically to pile more sand along the edges, but it was no use. With one mighty splash, a foamy wave surged forward, swallowing half the castle in seconds.

The family gasped, then burst into laughter as the once–towering structure slumped into a soggy heap. The seashell flags toppled, the moat disappeared, and one of the towers melted into a lopsided mound.

"Quick, save the king!" one of the kids shouted, holding up a tiny plastic figurine they had placed on top.

Other beachgoers clapped and cheered at the dramatic collapse, and soon the children were giggling as they stomped the remaining walls, turning the ruins into a giant sandy crater. Instead of disappointment, the family found joy in the moment. They spent the rest of the afternoon jumping waves, eating sandwiches, and laughing about how the ocean had "won the contest."

On the drive home, Grandma said, "I think that was our best castle yet." And everyone agreed, because the memory of its spectacular fall was far more lasting than the castle itself.

Singing the Wrong Words

The annual summer cookout at Uncle Joe's house always ended with music. After dinner, the family gathered on the porch, guitars came out, and voices rose together. Everyone looked forward to the sing–along, even if not all of them could carry a tune.

This year, Aunt Linda suggested they start with a popular old song that everyone knew by heart. At least, that was the plan.

Joe strummed the opening chords, and the group began to sing. But within seconds, it became clear that no one actually remembered the words. Aunt Linda confidently belted out one verse while Cousin Tom sang something completely different. The children made up their own silly rhymes, and Grandma clapped along, laughing too hard to even try.

"Wait, wait," Joe chuckled, pausing mid–strum. "How do none of us know the words?"

"Of course I know them," Aunt Linda said proudly, only to forget the next line and trail off.

Laughter filled the porch. Someone shouted, "Just keep going!" So they did, each person inventing lyrics on the spot. Instead of the original verses, the song turned into a hilarious mix of nonsense about hamburgers, sunscreen, and Uncle Joe's lopsided lawn chair.

By the second chorus, even the neighbors had come outside, drawn by the commotion. Rather than complain, they joined in, adding their own playful verses. The porch shook with laughter and clapping as the song grew funnier with every line.

When the final chord rang out, the family collapsed into their chairs, wiping tears from their eyes. "That," said Cousin Tom, "was the greatest version of the song ever sung."

From then on, the wrong–lyrics sing–along became a tradition. No one bothered to look up the actual words. Instead, every summer the family gathered on the porch to reinvent the song, turning it into something new and ridiculous each time.

Grandma called it "our family anthem," and the neighbors agreed. What began as a simple mistake turned into a beloved ritual, proof that the best music is not about perfection but about the laughter it creates.

Slip on Stage at the Talent Show

Every spring, the local elementary school hosted a talent show, and the gymnasium filled with excited parents, proud teachers, and nervous children. That year, two brothers, Jack and Sam, decided to perform together. Jack would sing while Sam played a simple tune on the piano. They practiced for weeks in their living room, turning mistakes into laughter and cheering each other on.

When the big night arrived, the boys dressed in their nicest clothes and waited backstage with the other performers. The lights were bright, the crowd was buzzing, and the brothers whispered encouragement to each other.

At last, their names were called. Sam marched confidently to the piano, and Jack followed, holding the microphone with both hands. The music began, and Jack's voice rose strong and clear. The first verse went smoothly, and their parents smiled proudly from the front row.

Then it happened. As Jack took a step forward to add a bit of flair, his foot caught on the edge of the stage rug. He stumbled, arms flailing, and landed on the floor with a loud thump. The audience gasped, and Sam froze mid–note, his hands hovering over the piano keys.

For a moment, there was silence. Then Jack popped back up, grinning sheepishly. "Don't worry, folks," he announced into the microphone. "That was part of the act!"

Laughter rippled through the gym. Sam quickly picked up the tune again, and Jack jumped right back into the song as if nothing had happened. The crowd clapped along, now even more invested in the performance.

By the end, the brothers received thunderous applause, not only for their music but for handling the mishap with humor. The principal even gave them a special mention: "Best recovery of the night."

Back at home, their parents hugged them tightly. "You were wonderful," their mom said. "And Jack, that fall might have made you the star of the show." The boys laughed, replaying the moment over and over, exaggerating Jack's tumble until it became a comedy routine of its own. From then on, whenever anyone mentioned the school talent show, people remembered the slip, the laughter, and the brothers who turned an accident into a highlight.

The Camping Tent Collapse

The Johnson family had planned their first camping trip in years. Armed with a brand-new tent, sleeping bags, and enough marshmallows to last a week, they arrived at the campsite full of enthusiasm. The forest was alive with chirping crickets and the smell of pine needles, and everyone felt adventurous.

The trouble began the moment they tried to set up the tent. The instructions looked more like a puzzle than a guide. Mr. Johnson held one pole upright while Mrs. Johnson tried to connect another piece, but the poles kept slipping apart. Their teenage daughter rolled her eyes, muttering that even her phone charger was easier to assemble. The youngest son, meanwhile, chased squirrels with a flashlight, offering no help at all.

After what felt like hours of tugging and pushing, the tent finally stood. Crooked, but standing. They all cheered and crawled inside, proud of their work. They roasted hot dogs, told ghost stories, and listened to the wind rustle through the trees. The night seemed perfect.

Until midnight.

A sudden gust of wind swept through the campsite. The tent shivered, then leaned dramatically to one side. Mr. Johnson tried to hold it up from inside, but the poles gave way with a loud snap. In an instant, the whole tent collapsed like a giant blanket fort, burying the family in nylon and zippers.

From the outside, it looked like a giant turtle had landed on the ground. Inside, the family struggled to untangle themselves, bumping heads and laughing so hard they could barely breathe. Mrs. Johnson kept insisting she had found the "door," but it turned out to be a mesh pocket. Their daughter recorded the chaos on her phone, vowing to post it online as soon as they had signal.

Finally, they wriggled out, hair sticking up and pajamas covered in grass. It was too late and too tiring to rebuild the tent, so they spread their sleeping bags under the open sky. The stars glittered above, brighter than any city light.

"This is better than the tent anyway," the youngest said, pointing at a shooting star.

They all agreed. What started as a disaster turned into the highlight of the trip. Wrapped in blankets, the Johnsons fell asleep together under the endless night sky, realizing that sometimes the best memories come when plans collapse—literally.

Tangled Up in Fishing Lines

The Harris family decided to spend a sunny Saturday morning at the lake. Armed with fishing poles, a cooler full of sandwiches, and plenty of optimism, they claimed a quiet spot on the dock. The water sparkled, and the gentle sound of waves against the wood made everything feel peaceful.

At least until they opened the tackle box.

Grandpa Harris, convinced he was the family's master fisherman, handed out hooks and lines with all the seriousness of a general preparing for battle. The problem was that no one in the family actually remembered how to fish properly. Dad tried to tie a knot that immediately slipped loose, Mom struggled to put bait on the hook, and the kids were more interested in seeing who could swing their fishing rod the highest.

Within minutes, chaos bloomed. Every time one of them cast a line, it landed exactly where it shouldn't. Mom's hook snagged the picnic basket, Dad's line wrapped itself around a chair leg, and one of the kids somehow managed to reel in Grandpa's hat.

"Hey! That's my lucky cap!" Grandpa shouted, trying to grab it back while everyone laughed.

The more they tried to untangle the mess, the worse it got. Lines crossed, hooks caught on sleeves, and at one point Dad nearly toppled into the lake while pulling at a particularly stubborn knot. A family of ducks floated by, quacking noisily, as if mocking the spectacle.

Finally, after what felt like an hour, they had created one enormous ball of fishing line. The poles were useless, and not a single fish had been caught. Instead of giving up, they spread out the picnic and watched the sun dance across the water. Grandpa wore his hat again, slightly bent from the rescue operation, and announced that fishing was overrated anyway.

As they bit into sandwiches, the kids teased their parents about their "legendary fishing skills." Laughter echoed across the dock, loud enough to startle the ducks into flight.

No one cared that they hadn't caught a thing. The day was already perfect. The tangled lines would be remembered as the funniest part of the trip, proof that sometimes the best catch isn't fish at all, but the memories made together.

Costume Fail at the Party

The Parker family was buzzing with excitement on the evening of the neighborhood carnival. Eight-year-old Emma had begged her mother to make her a fairy princess costume. She imagined ribbons, glitter, and flowing fabric that would shimmer under the lights. Mrs. Parker spent several evenings at the sewing machine, carefully stitching sparkles into the skirt and attaching tiny bells that chimed with every step.

When the big night arrived, Emma slipped into her costume and twirled in front of the mirror. Her eyes sparkled as much as the sequins on her dress. "I look magical," she said proudly. Her family applauded, and her older brother teased that she might float away if she twirled too fast.

At the community center, Emma paraded around with confidence. She posed for pictures, jingled her little bells, and told her friends she was sure to win the costume contest. Everything went smoothly until she reached for a slice of cake at the refreshment table. A loud rip echoed through the room. Her skirt had caught on a chair leg and torn nearly in half.

For a brief second, Emma froze in shock. A room full of eyes turned toward her. Then she surprised everyone by bursting out laughing. "Looks like I'm half fairy and half regular kid," she joked. The tension melted instantly, and soon the room filled with laughter and cheers.

Determined not to let the mishap ruin her evening, Emma improvised. She grabbed a colorful tablecloth and tied it around her shoulders like a cape. A balloon artist quickly twisted a crown for her, and her brother pinned one of the bells to her shirt. The transformation was complete. She was no longer a fairy princess but something entirely new: the Queen of Improv.

When the judges announced the winners, the crowd chanted Emma's name. To everyone's delight, her inventive costume earned her the prize for Most Original. She marched proudly onto the stage with her balloon crown wobbling and her cape fluttering behind her. The audience clapped and laughed until their cheeks hurt.

On the way home, Emma cuddled her prize ribbon and said, "Next year, let's make another costume, but it has to rip so I can win again." Her parents chuckled, knowing that the memory of that night would be retold at every carnival for years to come.

When April Fools Backfires

April first arrived with sunshine and mischief in the air. In the Miller household, April Fool's Day had always been a tradition filled with playful tricks. This year, twelve-year-old Max was determined to outsmart the entire family. He whispered his plan to his sister, who agreed to help him set the stage.

The idea seemed foolproof. Max poured apple juice into a bottle labeled "iced tea" and placed it in the fridge, hoping to trick his father. He also taped a piece of paper under the computer mouse so it would not work, targeting his mother. Finally, he stuffed cotton into his grandfather's slippers, sure that the old man would stumble when he tried them on. Max was certain this year's pranks would go down in family history.

Morning arrived and the family gathered in the kitchen. Mr. Miller reached for the fridge, spotted the bottle, and poured himself a glass. Max held his breath, waiting for the confusion. His father took a sip, paused for a moment, and then said calmly, "Thanks, son, I was hoping for apple juice this morning." Max's jaw dropped while the rest of the family chuckled.

Next came his mother. She sat at the computer and tried to move the mouse. After a few failed attempts she leaned back and smiled. "Nice try, Max. I used to play the same trick on my brothers." Max groaned, realizing his second prank had also failed.

Finally, Grandpa shuffled into the living room and slipped on his slippers. Instead of stumbling, he grinned and said, "Ah, extra cushioning. My feet have never felt so comfortable." The room erupted in laughter.

Max crossed his arms, defeated. "Nothing worked. Not one prank."

His sister, who had quietly been watching, stood up with a mischievous grin. "That's because I told them all about your plan yesterday." The room fell silent for a moment before bursting into laughter again. Max's elaborate April Fool's scheme had been sabotaged by his own teammate.

In the end, the joke was on him. But as he laughed along with everyone else, Max admitted it had been the funniest April Fool's Day yet.

Salt Instead of Sugar

On a quiet Sunday afternoon, Mrs. Thompson decided to bake a cake for her grandchildren. She pulled out her old recipe book, its pages smudged with flour and memories, and set her glasses on the counter. Unfortunately, she forgot to put them on.

She skimmed the faded handwriting, convinced she knew the instructions by heart. "One cup of salt," she read aloud with confidence. Without hesitation, she scooped a heaping cup of white crystals and poured it into the mixing bowl. The sugar jar sat nearby, ignored and forgotten.

As the oven warmed, the kitchen filled with the familiar scent of baking, though something seemed slightly off. Still, she carried on, humming happily as she prepared frosting. When the timer dinged, she proudly pulled out a golden, fluffy cake. It looked perfect, and she couldn't wait to surprise her family.

Her grandchildren burst into the kitchen, eager for dessert. Plates were handed out, slices cut, and forks raised in unison. The first bite brought an immediate reaction. Faces twisted, eyes bulged, and one grandson sputtered, "Grandma, this is the saltiest cake in the world!"

Mrs. Thompson took a bite herself and nearly laughed out the mouthful. The cake was inedible, but the moment was priceless. Her daughter gently pointed to the recipe card. "It says one cup of sugar, not salt." Everyone erupted into giggles as Grandma buried her face in her hands.

Instead of letting the failure ruin the afternoon, they turned it into a comedy show. The children dared each other to take tiny bites of the salty sponge, reacting with exaggerated expressions and dramatic groans. Grandpa even pretended it was delicious, taking a big forkful and declaring it "a new family delicacy."

The ruined dessert quickly became the highlight of the day. They ended up making sundaes with ice cream from the freezer while the salty cake sat proudly in the center of the table as a trophy of the funniest baking disaster yet.

From that day on, the family jokingly referred to the incident whenever someone cooked. "Remember to read the recipe," Grandma would say with a wink. The misread cake became a legend, proof that sometimes the sweetest memories come from mistakes.

Shopping List for Homework

Ten-year-old Daniel sat at the kitchen table late Sunday evening, finishing what he thought was his math homework. His mother had left the grocery list beside him, and in the shuffle of papers he mistakenly tucked it into his backpack. Tired but proud of himself, he zipped everything up and went to bed without noticing the mix-up.

The next morning, Daniel marched into class ready to hand in his work. His teacher, Mrs. Carter, collected the assignments one by one. When she reached Daniel's desk, he smiled and placed his paper on top of the pile, completely unaware of what was written on it.

Later that day, Mrs. Carter began grading during her lunch break. She opened Daniel's folder and blinked in surprise. Instead of math problems neatly solved, she found a list scrawled in his handwriting: "Milk, bread, bananas, chicken, dog food, and one large jar of pickles." At the bottom he had added, "Cookies, please," as if it were part of the assignment.

Mrs. Carter could not help laughing. She carried the paper back to class and held it up. "Daniel, I think your homework is a little… unusual." The class turned to look as Daniel's face turned bright red.

When she read the list aloud, the room erupted with laughter. His classmates shouted suggestions, adding their own imaginary items like "chocolate fountains" and "a pony." Daniel buried his head in his arms but soon started laughing too.

Instead of scolding him, Mrs. Carter gave him a playful smile. "Daniel, I'm afraid I cannot grade your grocery skills, but I'll give you an A plus in shopping." She pinned the list to the classroom bulletin board under the title "Most Original Homework of the Year."

Daniel went home that afternoon with a story that spread quickly through the neighborhood. Parents chuckled when they heard about the mix-up, and his mother proudly declared that at least he remembered all the things she needed from the store.

From then on, Daniel double-checked every paper before handing it in. Still, the Wrong Homework Assignment became a family legend, retold at every school gathering as proof that even mistakes can earn a smile.

The Neighborhood Parade Giggle

Every summer, the little town of Willow Creek held a neighborhood parade. It was never a grand event with floats or marching bands, but rather a cheerful gathering of families, kids on decorated bicycles, and neighbors who played instruments for fun. This year, everyone was especially excited because the local brass group had promised to perform along the route.

On the morning of the parade, children taped streamers to their handlebars and tied balloons to wagons. Parents lined the sidewalks with folding chairs while grandparents waved from porches. The brass group gathered at the front, polishing their instruments and warming up with enthusiasm. Spirits were high as the crowd clapped to signal the start.

At first, everything went smoothly. The trumpets played a bright melody, the trombones followed with gusto, and the drummers kept a steady beat. But after the second block, something shifted. One trumpet player started in on a completely different tune, convinced it was the right one. The trombones tried to follow, but half of them stuck with the original song. The drummers, confused, picked up a new rhythm entirely.

Within minutes, the once orderly parade band sounded like three different groups competing for attention. The audience tilted their heads, unsure whether to laugh or cover their ears. Then a little boy in the crowd shouted, "Play louder!" and the musicians obliged. The result was a glorious cacophony of mismatched notes and clashing beats.

Instead of disappointment, the chaos brought laughter. Parents chuckled, children giggled, and even the musicians began to smile through their off-key performance. Some of them leaned into the silliness, exaggerating their playing as if it were a comedy act. The crowd clapped along, turning the parade into an impromptu street festival.

By the time the band reached the park, no one cared about the missed notes. People were laughing so hard that tears rolled down their cheeks. Someone declared it the funniest parade Willow Creek had ever seen. The brass group took a bow, proud of their unintentional comedy show.

From that day on, neighbors fondly remembered the year when the parade turned into a giggle-fest. What was supposed to be a polished performance became a story told again and again, proof that joy often comes from the most unexpected mistakes.

Singing with the Frogs

On a warm summer evening, the kids of Maple Street decided to gather at the small pond near the edge of the woods. It was their favorite spot, a place where dragonflies hovered over the water and fireflies sparkled in the tall grass. They spread out blankets, shared snacks, and waited for the sunset to paint the sky in shades of pink and orange.

As the last light faded, the first croaks began. One frog gave a low rumble near the reeds. Another answered from the opposite bank. Soon the entire pond erupted with sound, a chorus of croaks, ribbits, and deep, throaty calls that echoed through the night air.

The children listened in awe. It was so loud they had to lean close just to talk. Then one of the boys cupped his hands around his mouth and tried to imitate the frogs. His "ribbit" was so exaggerated that everyone burst into laughter. Not to be outdone, the others joined in. Within minutes, the group was croaking and chirping along, creating their own version of a frog choir.

They began experimenting with rhythms, some croaking fast, others stretching out long notes. The frogs seemed to respond, as if joining the playful contest. The children laughed until their sides ached, doubling over whenever someone's voice cracked or came out more like a squeaky duck than a frog.

Even the adults sitting nearby couldn't resist. A grandmother gave her best croak, surprising everyone with how realistic it sounded. That only fueled the fun, and soon the whole gathering was echoing the pond in a comical back-and-forth of human and frog voices.

When the laughter finally quieted, they lay back on their blankets, watching the stars emerge above the trees. The frogs continued their song, steady and strong, as if proud of their unexpected duet with the neighborhood children.

From that night on, the kids called themselves the Frog Choir. Every summer evening, they returned to the pond, eager to listen, laugh, and join in. It became a tradition that bound them together, a reminder that sometimes the best music is the one made out of joy and silliness.

The pond never sounded quite the same again, and for the families of Maple Street, that chorus of frogs and giggles became one of their happiest memories.

The Hearing Aid Surprise

Sunday dinners at the Peterson household were always lively, filled with chatter, clinking dishes, and plenty of laughter. Grandpa Harold, with his booming personality, usually sat at the head of the table, telling jokes and stories that had the whole family in stitches. This particular evening, however, something seemed different.

Every time someone spoke, Grandpa responded with an answer that didn't quite fit. When his daughter mentioned that the chicken was a little dry, he replied, "Yes, the weather has been very sunny." The grandchildren looked at each other, trying to hold back their giggles.

Later, when his son-in-law asked about the baseball game, Grandpa nodded solemnly and said, "Oh yes, I agree, the curtains do need washing." The table erupted with laughter, though Grandpa smiled proudly, convinced his wit was sharper than ever.

As the evening went on, the mismatched replies grew funnier. His granddaughter explained how she had won first place in the school spelling bee. Grandpa clapped and announced, "That's wonderful, I also enjoy strawberry pie." The family laughed so hard they had to put down their forks.

Finally, his wife leaned over and noticed something. "Harold," she said gently, "your hearing aid isn't even turned on." Grandpa blinked in surprise, reached to his ear, and realized she was right. He had spent the entire evening answering conversations without hearing a word.

Instead of being embarrassed, Grandpa threw back his head and laughed louder than anyone else. "Well," he declared, "I suppose I'm funnier when I don't hear a thing."

The rest of the family cheered, and the grandchildren crowned him "Comedian of the Year" on the spot. From that day forward, whenever Grandpa gave an odd answer, they jokingly asked if his hearing aid was off again.

What could have been a small mishap turned into a treasured family story. Grandpa's hearing aid surprise became part of the family's lore, retold at reunions and dinners with the same laughter that filled the room that Sunday evening.

Calling the Wrong Old Friend

The community hall was buzzing with chatter as old classmates reunited after decades apart. Tables were decorated with photo albums, name tags, and bowls of candy meant to break the ice. Mrs. Greene, who had not seen many of her classmates since graduation, walked in with excitement and a little nervousness.

Almost immediately, she spotted a tall gentleman near the refreshment table. Convinced she recognized him as Peter, a boy she had sat next to in English class, she hurried over. "Peter, it's so good to see you again!" she exclaimed, patting him warmly on the shoulder.

The man smiled politely. "Well, it's good to see you too," he said, though his tone carried a hint of hesitation.

Throughout the evening, Mrs. Greene kept calling him Peter. She introduced him to others with the same confidence. "Do you remember Peter? He used to draw cartoons on the back of his homework," she announced, laughing as if the memories were crystal clear. The gentleman nodded along, chuckling softly, though never actually confirming her story.

As the night wore on, her stories grew more elaborate. She recounted the time Peter supposedly spilled ink on the teacher's desk and the way he once tried to sing in the school choir. Each tale earned laughter from the group, and the man simply went along, enjoying the attention.

Finally, near the end of the evening, Mrs. Greene noticed his name tag. It clearly read "Michael." She frowned and asked, "Why does your tag say Michael? Did they make a mistake?"

At that, the man burst out laughing. "No mistake," he admitted. "My name really is Michael. I didn't even go to this school. I just came with my wife, who's over there catching up with her class."

For a moment, Mrs. Greene was speechless. Then she doubled over in laughter, joined by everyone around them. What could have been embarrassing turned into the funniest moment of the reunion.

From then on, she and Michael became fast friends, joking that he was her "fake classmate." The story of the wrong name became one of the most retold highlights of the evening, proving that even mix-ups can create new connections.

Dentures on the Loose

It was family game night at the Martinez household, and the living room was filled with laughter, snacks, and playful competition. Grandpa Joe was in his element, telling jokes between turns of cards and making everyone laugh so hard they could barely focus on the game.

As the evening went on, Grandpa launched into one of his favorite long stories, the kind that always had a big punchline. He leaned forward, gesturing dramatically, his voice rising as he built suspense. Just as he reached the funniest part, something unexpected happened. His dentures slipped out with a small clatter onto the table.

For a split second, the room went silent. Then chaos erupted. The grandchildren shrieked with laughter, covering their mouths while pointing at the table. His daughter tried to stifle her giggles but ended up laughing so hard that tears rolled down her cheeks. Even Grandpa Joe looked stunned for a moment, then burst into the loudest laugh of them all.

Not willing to let the moment pass, he picked up the dentures and made them "talk," pretending they had stolen the punchline of his joke. "Don't blame me," he said in a silly voice, moving the teeth like a puppet. "I couldn't hold on any longer!" The family howled with laughter, nearly falling out of their chairs.

From that point on, the game was forgotten. Everyone begged Grandpa to make the dentures perform more tricks. He obliged, giving them different voices, singing a few notes, and even pretending they were auditioning for a comedy show. The living room turned into an impromptu stage, and the dentures became the star of the evening.

When the laughter finally died down, Grandpa wiped his eyes and said, "Well, I guess I've found my new sidekick." The grandchildren quickly declared the dentures the official mascot of family game night.

What began as an awkward accident became one of the funniest memories the family ever shared. Every game night afterward, someone would inevitably ask, "Are the dentures joining us tonight?" and the whole room would erupt in laughter again.

Grandpa Joe never minded the teasing. In fact, he leaned into the joke, proud that his unexpected mishap had brought the family even closer together.

Chasing the Runaway Cane

Mr. Wallace loved his daily walks through the neighborhood. At eighty years old, he relied on a sturdy wooden cane that had accompanied him for years. One breezy afternoon, he paused at the top of a small hill to chat with a neighbor. Without noticing, he leaned his cane against a garden wall while he talked about the weather and the latest news.

As the conversation carried on, a gust of wind nudged the cane, and it began to slide. Slowly at first, then faster, it picked up speed down the gentle slope of the sidewalk. By the time Mr. Wallace turned around, it was already rolling toward the bottom of the hill.

"Stop that cane!" he shouted with surprising energy. His neighbor burst into laughter as Mr. Wallace broke into an unexpected sprint. The sight was comical: an elderly man chasing a runaway cane that seemed to have developed a mind of its own.

Children playing nearby joined in the fun, running alongside the cane as if it were part of a race. One boy even cheered, "Go, cane, go!" Neighbors stepped out of their houses to watch, clapping and laughing at the spectacle.

The cane finally slowed near a patch of grass, but not before Mr. Wallace lunged forward and grabbed it with triumphant flair. He raised it high in the air like a trophy while everyone applauded. Breathless but grinning, he declared, "Fastest race I've run in years!"

Someone handed him a bottle of water, and the children asked if they could race with him again. Mr. Wallace chuckled and said, "Only if my cane agrees." The crowd erupted once more, delighted by his humor.

From that day, the neighborhood jokingly crowned him the champion of the "Cane Dash." On warm afternoons, the children would tease him by pretending to set the cane rolling again, and Mr. Wallace would play along, pretending to stretch like an athlete before the chase.

What began as a simple accident became a joyful memory for the whole street. For Mr. Wallace, it was proof that laughter and a little speed could still surprise everyone, including himself.

Sock Skating in the Hallway

The Carter family had hardwood floors that gleamed after every cleaning. They looked beautiful, but they also had a secret hazard. One winter morning, twelve-year-old Lily discovered it by accident when she came running down the hallway in her favorite fuzzy socks. Instead of stopping at the kitchen door, she slid halfway across the floor and landed with a surprised squeal.

Her brother burst out laughing. "Do it again!" he shouted. Lily, brushing herself off, grinned and took another running start. Soon she was sliding like a professional skater, arms spread wide for balance. Her mother walked in just in time to see Lily zoom past and shook her head with a smile.

Before long, the whole family joined in. Dad grabbed a pair of thick socks and proved he could glide even farther than the kids. Their mother, not wanting to be left out, shuffled quickly and slid a few feet, laughing so hard she nearly toppled over. Even Grandma, visiting for the weekend, decided to give it a try. With surprising speed, she shot down the hall, and everyone cheered as if she had just won a medal.

The hallway turned into their unofficial skating rink. They marked start and finish lines with pieces of tape, keeping score of who could slide the farthest. Each attempt brought more laughter, especially when someone lost balance and flopped onto the floor in a dramatic spin. The dog barked excitedly, chasing after whoever was sliding, as if trying to join the game.

By the afternoon, the family had created a full competition complete with rounds and playful commentary. Grandpa served as the announcer, declaring Lily "the queen of the socks" and Dad "the champion of style." When Grandma took the title for longest slide, everyone erupted in applause.

At the end of the day, they collapsed on the couch, cheeks sore from laughing. The polished floor bore a few extra scuff marks, but nobody cared.

From then on, whenever the family wore socks on the hardwood floor, someone would inevitably shout, "Race time!" and the sliding would begin again. What started as a simple slip turned into one of the most beloved traditions in the Carter household.

Looking for Glasses Already Worn

Mrs. Collins prided herself on being organized. She kept her kitchen spotless, her living room tidy, and her knitting basket neatly arranged by color. But one thing seemed to vanish from her life on a regular basis: her glasses.

One quiet afternoon, she was preparing to read a new mystery novel. She reached for her glasses on the side table, but they weren't there. She checked the kitchen counter, the mantel, and even the windowsill, but they had disappeared again. With a sigh, she began the all-too-familiar hunt.

She searched the couch cushions, convinced they had slipped between them. She rummaged through her purse, finding everything from old receipts to peppermints, but no glasses. Growing frustrated, she called out to her husband. "Harold, have you seen my glasses?"

Harold looked up from his crossword puzzle and studied her for a moment. He grinned but said nothing.

Mrs. Collins continued her quest. She peeked inside the refrigerator, just in case she had set them down while putting away groceries. She opened drawers in the bedroom, checked the bathroom shelf, and even looked under the dog's blanket. Still no sign.

Finally, she marched back into the living room with her hands on her hips. "This is ridiculous. They've vanished into thin air."

Harold chuckled and pointed at her head. "You mean those glasses?"

Mrs. Collins froze. Sure enough, the glasses were perched right on top of her hair, exactly where she had placed them an hour earlier.

For a moment she felt embarrassed, but then she burst into laughter. "Well," she admitted, "at least I kept them in a safe place."

The story became an instant favorite among family and friends. Her grandchildren teased her by pretending to search for their own glasses, only to reveal them sitting on their foreheads. Even Harold joined in the fun, occasionally asking, "Looking for something, dear?" whenever she walked around the house.

From then on, the phrase "check your head" became a running joke in the Collins household. What started as a frustrating search turned into one of their happiest and most repeated family memories.

Bingo Numbers All Wrong

The community center buzzed with excitement on Friday night. Bingo night was a weekly tradition, and the hall filled quickly with neighbors eager for laughter, prizes, and the thrill of marking numbers on their cards. Mr. Lawson, a cheerful retiree with a booming voice, always claimed the same seat near the front, convinced it brought him good luck.

This evening began like any other. The caller shouted out numbers, and players leaned over their cards with intense focus. "B nine," echoed through the microphone. People dabbed their cards with brightly colored markers. "G forty-eight," the caller continued. The room was filled with murmurs and the soft thud of markers tapping paper.

Mr. Lawson, however, seemed more enthusiastic than usual. Each time a number was called, he marked his card with exaggerated flair. "Got it!" he announced, smiling proudly at the people around him. His neighbors raised their eyebrows, surprised at his streak of luck.

By the time the caller reached the mid-game, Mr. Lawson's card was nearly full. He leaned back with satisfaction, ready to win big. Then the caller announced, "N thirty-one." Mr. Lawson jumped to his feet and shouted, "Bingo!" His voice echoed across the hall.

The room fell silent. The caller walked over, ready to check his card. But when she leaned down, she frowned. "Mr. Lawson, your numbers don't match at all."

Everyone craned their necks as the mistake became clear. Instead of following the caller's announcements, Mr. Lawson had been marking random numbers across his card, creating a colorful but completely incorrect masterpiece.

For a second, Mr. Lawson looked stunned. Then he burst into hearty laughter, clutching his belly as tears streamed down his cheeks. The crowd joined in, clapping and cheering. Someone joked that he had invented a new game called "Creative Bingo."

The caller, still smiling, handed him a small prize anyway. "For originality," she said, as the room erupted once more in laughter. Mr. Lawson bowed dramatically, holding up his card like it was a work of art.

From that night on, the story of the Bingo Card Blunder was retold at every gathering. Mr. Lawson's mistake had given the entire community a memory far more valuable than any prize.

Two Trips, Same Shopping List

Mr. and Mrs. Turner had been married for more than forty years, and they knew each other's habits almost too well. One Saturday morning, Mrs. Turner announced she was heading to the supermarket. At the same time, Mr. Turner decided to take a stroll and thought he might as well do the grocery shopping too. Neither mentioned their plans, assuming the other would stay home.

At the store, Mrs. Turner carefully filled her cart with the week's essentials: milk, bread, eggs, fruit, and her husband's favorite cookies. Meanwhile, in another aisle, Mr. Turner was selecting the exact same items, even down to the cookies. Without realizing it, they both checked out, packed their groceries into identical brown bags, and drove home separately.

Mrs. Turner arrived first. She unpacked her bags, humming happily as she arranged everything neatly in the kitchen. A few minutes later, the front door opened and Mr. Turner walked in with his own load of bags.

She blinked in confusion. "Why are you carrying groceries? I already went this morning."

Mr. Turner looked at the counter, where identical items were already lined up. "What do you mean you went? I just bought all of this!"

They both burst into laughter as they compared their hauls. Two cartons of milk, two loaves of bread, four dozen eggs, and an impressive mountain of cookies covered the counter. Even the fruit matched perfectly.

Their grandchildren, visiting later that afternoon, could not stop laughing when they saw the overflowing pantry. "Are you opening a grocery store?" one of them teased. Mr. Turner chuckled and said, "At least we'll never run out of snacks."

The family spent the rest of the weekend joking about the great grocery duplication. Meals became playful challenges to see how many eggs or cookies they could use at once. Mrs. Turner baked pies and cakes, while Mr. Turner declared himself in charge of milkshakes.

By the end of the week, the duplicate shopping trip had turned into a fond memory and a story retold many times. Whenever they headed out for errands afterward, they made sure to check with each other first. Still, the grandchildren secretly hoped they might forget again, just for another round of laughter.

Wallet Found in the Freezer

Mr. Bradley was known in his family for being forgetful. He often misplaced his reading glasses, left the television remote in the refrigerator, and once even spent an afternoon searching for his phone while it was in his pocket. But the day he lost his wallet topped them all.

It began on a chilly Saturday morning. He reached for his coat pocket before heading out to the market and froze. The wallet was gone. Panic set in as he patted his pockets, checked the hall table, and rifled through drawers. Mrs. Bradley joined the search, lifting couch cushions and peering under chairs. Their grandchildren pitched in too, crawling on the floor in hopes of finding the missing treasure.

Hours passed, and frustration grew. Mr. Bradley muttered about thieves and conspiracies, while his wife shook her head. "It has to be somewhere in the house," she insisted. The grandchildren suggested retracing every step of his morning. They searched the garden shed, the laundry room, and even the mailbox. Still nothing.

By late afternoon, everyone was exhausted. Mr. Bradley slumped into the kitchen chair with a heavy sigh. "It's hopeless," he said. He opened the freezer to grab some ice for his drink and suddenly stopped. There, tucked neatly between a loaf of bread and a bag of frozen peas, sat his leather wallet.

The room went silent for a beat, then erupted in laughter. Mrs. Bradley laughed so hard she had to hold onto the counter. "Why on earth would you put it in there?" she asked through tears of amusement.

Mr. Bradley scratched his head sheepishly. "I must have been holding it while I was putting away groceries. Guess I thought the wallet needed to stay fresh too."

The grandchildren cheered as if he had just performed a magic trick. For weeks afterward, the family teased him about his "frozen assets." At every gathering, someone would ask, "Grandpa, is your wallet still on ice?"

Though he felt a little embarrassed, Mr. Bradley admitted it was one of the funniest mistakes he had ever made. The missing wallet became a legendary story in the Bradley household, proof that sometimes the best memories come from the coldest surprises.

Lost but Laughing on the Road

The Petersons loved taking road trips. Every summer they packed the car with snacks, maps, and a playlist of old songs that everyone could sing along to. This year, they set out to visit a famous landmark two hours away. Spirits were high as they drove along winding country roads, windows rolled down to let in the warm breeze.

Mr. Peterson proudly declared himself the navigator, even though his wife had gently suggested they use the GPS. "I know these roads like the back of my hand," he boasted. For a while, everything seemed fine. Rolling fields stretched out on either side, and the kids in the backseat played car games, shouting out animals they spotted along the way.

After an hour, Mrs. Peterson began to frown. "Are you sure this is the right way?" she asked. The road had narrowed, and the signs no longer mentioned their destination. Mr. Peterson waved her concern aside. "Trust me, I've got it under control."

Another half hour passed before they entered a small village they had never seen before. Instead of tourist buses and souvenir shops, they found a quaint square with a bakery, a flower stall, and a group of locals setting up for what looked like a festival. Curious, the family parked the car and stepped out.

Almost immediately, they were greeted by a cheerful woman offering fresh pastries. A band started tuning instruments nearby, and colorful banners fluttered overhead. The Petersons had stumbled upon the village's annual summer celebration.

The children raced to join the games in the square, while Mrs. Peterson sampled homemade jam. Mr. Peterson, trying to save face, announced, "Of course I knew this was here. It was part of the plan." His family laughed, knowing better but enjoying the day too much to argue.

They spent hours dancing, tasting food, and making new friends. When the sun began to set, they finally got back into the car, tired but happy. The landmark they had set out to see no longer mattered.

On the drive home, Mrs. Peterson smiled. "That wrong turn might have been the best decision you ever made." Mr. Peterson grinned and replied, "See, I told you I knew where we were going."

The road trip that began with confusion ended as one of the family's favorite adventures, remembered not for the destination but for the unexpected joy found along the way.

Christmas Lights in a Knot

The Anderson family always took holiday decorating seriously. Every December, they transformed their home into the brightest house on the block. Boxes of ornaments, wreaths, and lights came down from the attic, and everyone pitched in to create a festive wonderland.

This year, the task of untangling the outdoor Christmas lights fell to Mr. Anderson and his teenage son, Mark. The two dragged out a box stuffed with strands that had been hastily packed away the year before. When they pulled the first string, it came out as one massive knot, twisted so tightly it looked like a glowing ball of spaghetti.

"Who packed these up?" Mr. Anderson groaned.

"You did," Mark replied with a grin.

The two sat on the porch, trying to separate the strands. They pulled, tugged, and shook the lights, but the knots only grew tighter. At one point, Mark had the string wrapped around his arm, while Mr. Anderson managed to loop it around his ankle. Their attempts to free themselves looked less like decorating and more like a comedy show.

Mrs. Anderson came outside carrying mugs of hot cocoa and burst out laughing at the sight of her husband and son wrestling with wires. "At this rate, the neighbors will think we're practicing a new dance routine," she teased.

After nearly an hour, they finally managed to spread the lights across the lawn. Triumph quickly faded when they plugged them in. Half the bulbs flickered weakly, while the rest stayed dark. Mark shrugged. "Maybe it's modern art."

Instead of giving up, they strung the tangled ball of lights onto the porch railing and draped the working section across the bushes. The final result looked far from professional, but it glowed brightly enough to bring cheer.

That evening, neighbors walked by and chuckled at the unusual display. One even commented, "I love your light sculpture. Very creative." The Andersons laughed, realizing their decorating disaster had accidentally turned into a neighborhood highlight.

From then on, the family embraced the tradition. Every year, they deliberately hung at least one knotted strand, calling it the "Anderson masterpiece." What began as a frustrating mess became a story of laughter and togetherness, shining as brightly as any perfectly strung lights.

The Turkey That Wouldn't Fit the Oven

Thanksgiving morning dawned with the smell of spices and the sound of holiday music in the Miller household. Mrs. Miller had been planning the meal for weeks, determined to prepare the perfect feast for her children and grandchildren. The centerpiece of it all was a massive turkey, the largest she had ever bought.

When Mr. Miller carried it into the kitchen, the bird barely fit on the counter. "Are we feeding the entire neighborhood?" he joked, raising his eyebrows at its size.

Mrs. Miller brushed off the comment. "Bigger is better. Everyone will have plenty of leftovers." She rubbed the turkey with herbs and butter, humming cheerfully as the family gathered around to watch.

The cheer faded quickly when it came time to slide the turkey into the oven. No matter how they turned it, twisted it, or pushed, the bird refused to fit. One wing stuck out when they tried lengthwise, and the legs bumped the oven door when they tried sideways.

The grandchildren giggled as Grandpa suggested using a hammer to "reshape it." Mrs. Miller gave him a look but could not help laughing herself when he mimed flattening it like a pancake.

For the next half hour, the family tried every idea. Someone suggested removing the oven rack, another thought about sawing the turkey in half, and one grandchild whispered that maybe they should just put it on the grill outside. Finally, Mr. Miller fetched a sharp knife and carefully cut the turkey into two large pieces.

The solution worked. They roasted one half at a time, keeping the rest warm in the meantime. Though it was not the elegant presentation Mrs. Miller had imagined, the aroma filled the kitchen, and soon the table was piled high with juicy slices.

When they sat down to eat, the family toasted to their resourcefulness. The grandchildren declared it the funniest Thanksgiving ever, and someone suggested that next year they should just buy two smaller turkeys. Mrs. Miller shook her head with a smile. "Never again," she said, though everyone doubted she meant it.

The story of the turkey that would not fit the oven became a favorite holiday tale, retold every year with more laughter and embellishment.

Valentine's Card to the Wrong Man

Valentine's Day was always a cheerful occasion in the Sanders household. Mr. Sanders made it a tradition to bring home flowers for his wife, while she often surprised him with his favorite chocolates. This year, Mrs. Sanders decided to go the extra mile and write a heartfelt card to slip into his jacket pocket before he left for work.

She carefully chose her words, filling the card with sweet memories and affectionate notes. With a smile, she sealed the envelope, addressed simply with the word "Darling," and placed it by the front door where her husband usually kept his coat.

The morning was busy. Children rushed to gather schoolbags, the dog barked for attention, and the phone rang with a neighbor's question about borrowing sugar. In the commotion, Mrs. Sanders accidentally slipped the card into the wrong jacket. Instead of her husband's, it went into Mr. Peterson's coat, their friendly neighbor who had stopped by to drop off a tool.

Later that day, Mr. Peterson reached into his pocket and discovered the envelope. Curious, he opened it—and nearly dropped it in shock when he read the affectionate message inside. His cheeks turned red, and he quickly knocked on the Sanders' door, card in hand.

Mrs. Sanders gasped when she realized what had happened. Before she could apologize, Mr. Sanders walked into the room, raising an eyebrow at the sight of his neighbor holding the Valentine's card. "Well," he said with a grin, "I didn't expect to have competition this year."

The three of them burst into laughter, and soon the story spread through the neighborhood. The children found it hilarious and teased their mother, calling Mr. Peterson her "secret Valentine."

To make up for the mix-up, Mrs. Sanders baked a batch of heart-shaped cookies and delivered a plate to the Petersons, who accepted them with good humor. Mr. Peterson even joked, "I'll treasure the card forever. It's the sweetest Valentine I've ever received."

From then on, every February, the families shared a laugh about the famous Valentine's Day mix-up, proving that even small accidents can turn into stories that bring people closer together.

Melted Chocolate Egg Hunt

Easter Sunday dawned warm and sunny, perfect for the annual egg hunt at Grandma Wilson's house. The grandchildren arrived with baskets in hand, eager to search the garden for the colorful eggs she had hidden. This year, she had filled dozens of chocolate eggs with small surprises inside, determined to outdo herself.

The children dashed into the yard, squealing with excitement as they spotted eggs tucked under bushes, nestled in flowerpots, and perched in the branches of the old oak tree. Their baskets quickly filled with shiny foil wrappers glinting in the sunlight. Laughter and shouts echoed through the neighborhood as they compared their treasures.

But after a while, the heat of the day began to take its toll. When little Emily unwrapped her first prize, she gasped. Instead of a solid egg, her hands were coated in gooey chocolate. "Grandma, my egg melted!" she cried.

Soon the other children discovered the same problem. One by one, they peeled back wrappers only to find squishy, misshapen blobs. Their fingers grew sticky, and their faces became smudged with chocolate as they tried to eat the melting treats.

The adults rushed to help, but the sight was too funny to ignore. Mr. Wilson chuckled as he handed out napkins, while Grandma covered her mouth to hide her laughter. "Well," she admitted, "I may have forgotten to think about the weather."

Instead of being upset, the children embraced the chaos. They licked their fingers, smeared chocolate on each other's noses, and declared it the best egg hunt ever. The melted eggs turned into a sticky but joyful mess, with everyone laughing as they tried to salvage the sweet prizes.

To rescue the day, Grandma brought out bowls and spoons. She scooped the melted chocolate into dishes, topping it with sprinkles and marshmallows. "There," she said proudly, "Easter sundaes." The children cheered, delighted with their unexpected dessert.

By evening, the garden was full of giggles and chocolate-covered smiles. What could have been a disaster turned into one of the most memorable Easter celebrations the family had ever shared.

From that year on, Grandma never forgot to hide a few eggs indoors as a backup. Still, the legend of the melted Easter eggs was retold every spring, always bringing back laughter as sweet as the chocolate itself.

Little Firework with Big Sparks

The Johnson family loved the Fourth of July. Every year they hosted a backyard barbecue with friends, neighbors, and enough food to feed an army. The kids looked forward to the evening most of all, when fireworks lit up the sky and sparklers were handed out to everyone.

This year, seven-year-old Tommy was especially excited. He had been waiting all day to wave his first sparkler. As the sun set and the grill cooled, the adults passed them out. The children gathered in a circle, squealing as the sparklers hissed to life, throwing off golden sparks.

Tommy gripped his sparkler tightly, his eyes wide with wonder. He spun in slow circles at first, drawing glowing shapes in the air. Then, caught up in the thrill, he began waving it faster and faster, like a tiny sword. The sparks flew higher, scattering dangerously close to the picnic table.

"Careful, Tommy!" his mother called, but he was too caught up in the excitement to notice. Suddenly, the sparkler fizzed wildly, and Tommy dashed toward his cousins with it still in his hand. The group screamed, half in fear and half in laughter, scattering across the yard like startled birds.

The adults rushed in, and Uncle Mike gently scooped Tommy up, plucking the sparkler from his grip. "Whoa there, little firecracker," he said with a chuckle. "You almost turned this into a fireworks show of your own."

Tommy looked sheepish for a moment, then broke into a grin. "Did you see how fast I was?" he asked proudly. His cousins burst out laughing, already teasing him by calling him "the human firework."

Once the sparks died down, the family gathered again, this time with stricter rules and sparklers only in calm, careful hands. Still, the incident became the highlight of the evening. The children re-enacted Tommy's wild dash, running around the yard with invisible sparklers while the adults laughed and shook their heads.

Later that night, as the sky exploded with dazzling fireworks, Tommy snuggled into his blanket and whispered, "I think I was brighter than those fireworks." His parents laughed softly, knowing the story of the sparkler scare would be told at every Independence Day party for years to come.

Twins in the Same Costume

The annual Halloween party at the community center was the highlight of autumn in Maplewood. Families arrived in elaborate costumes, from witches and ghosts to superheroes and clowns. The room was filled with laughter, music, and the rustle of candy wrappers.

Among the guests were Mr. and Mrs. Howard, who had decided to surprise everyone with a clever idea. They each dressed as a giant pumpkin, complete with bright orange suits and green leafy hats. They were sure their matching outfits would steal the show.

The surprise came when they walked through the door and spotted another couple across the room wearing the exact same costume. Mr. and Mrs. Bennett, longtime friends of the Howards, had also decided to dress as pumpkins. The two couples locked eyes and burst out laughing.

For the rest of the evening, the partygoers could not stop teasing them. "Which pumpkin is which?" someone joked. Children ran between the couples, pretending they were lost in a pumpkin patch. Even the host of the party joined in, suggesting a contest to see which pair wore it best.

At first, the Howards and the Bennetts posed for photos, showing off their round orange outfits. But soon the competition turned playful. They staged silly challenges, like rolling themselves across the dance floor and seeing who could wobble the most convincingly. The crowd roared with laughter, cheering for both sides.

When it came time to award prizes, the judges faced a dilemma. They whispered, argued, and finally gave up. "We can't decide," the announcer declared. "The prize for best costume goes to both pumpkin couples."

The hall erupted in applause as the Howards and the Bennetts took the stage together. Instead of competing, they linked arms and bowed as a united pumpkin patch. The children cheered, and cameras flashed as the moment was captured for the town newsletter.

On the way home, Mr. Howard chuckled. "Next year, we should coordinate ahead of time." Mrs. Bennett laughed. "Or maybe we should just keep the tradition and see who else turns into a pumpkin."

The Halloween costume confusion became a cherished memory in Maplewood, a story retold at every party. It proved that sometimes the best fun comes not from standing out, but from blending in perfectly with friends.

Celebrating Midnight Too Early

New Year's Eve was always a lively occasion in the Rivera household. Relatives gathered from near and far, crowding the living room with trays of food, clinking glasses, and plenty of noise. The children played with balloons while the adults debated resolutions and shared stories of the past year.

As midnight drew near, everyone turned their attention to the television. The famous countdown in Times Square was about to begin. Mr. Rivera adjusted the volume, and the family huddled together, ready to shout the numbers in unison.

The screen showed the sparkling ball glowing brightly. The announcer's voice boomed, "Ten, nine, eight..." Excitement filled the room as voices joined the countdown. But just as the family shouted "Happy New Year," something felt strange. The neighbors outside were still quiet. No fireworks, no cheering, only silence.

Confused, Mrs. Rivera glanced at the clock on the wall. It read eleven thirty. Somehow, they had been watching a broadcast from a different time zone. They had celebrated thirty minutes too early.

For a moment, the room was silent. Then laughter erupted. The children rolled on the floor, giggling at the mistake. Mr. Rivera threw his arms in the air and shouted, "We're trendsetters! First to celebrate!" His brother added, "We get two New Years this way—double the good luck!"

The family decided to make the most of it. They toasted with sparkling cider, danced to music, and then prepared to do it all again at the real midnight. When the second countdown finally arrived, they cheered even louder than before, blowing party horns and popping confetti as fireworks lit the sky outside.

The double celebration became a tradition. Every year after that, the Riveras held two countdowns—one early, one on time. Guests would tease them by asking, "Which New Year are we celebrating first?" The mistake that could have been embarrassing instead became a story that brought joy year after year.

That night, as the family finally settled down, Mrs. Rivera smiled and said, "Sometimes being wrong is more fun than being right." Everyone agreed, already looking forward to the next double New Year.

Runaway Birthday Balloons

The Parker family loved celebrating birthdays in style. When little Sophie turned six, her parents filled the backyard with decorations, a cake shaped like a castle, and dozens of bright balloons tied to chairs, tables, and fences. The yard shimmered with color as guests arrived carrying gifts and laughter.

Sophie's eyes sparkled when she saw the balloons dancing in the breeze. She ran from one to another, pointing out her favorites. "That one looks like a strawberry!" she squealed, hugging a red balloon with both arms.

As the party games began, the children raced around the yard while the balloons swayed above them. Everything was going perfectly until a sudden gust of wind swept through. Strings slipped loose, knots came undone, and in an instant half the balloons soared into the sky.

The children gasped, then broke into shrieks of excitement. "Catch them!" someone shouted. Dozens of little feet stampeded across the grass as the kids leapt and stretched their arms, trying to snatch the floating treasures. The balloons drifted higher, shimmering like jewels against the blue sky.

Sophie stood in the middle of the yard, her mouth wide open in surprise. Then she started to giggle. "Look, they're going to have their own party in the clouds!" she said. Her friends burst out laughing and joined her in waving goodbye to the runaway balloons.

The adults hurried to tie down the remaining decorations, but they too were laughing at the sight of children running after the colorful swarm. Even Grandma joined in, shaking her fist at the sky and joking that she wanted her balloon back.

When the excitement settled, Sophie received a special surprise. Her father handed her one balloon that had stayed behind, tied tightly to the back of her chair. "This one wanted to stay with you," he said. Sophie hugged it close, proud to have the lone survivor of the great balloon escape.

The story became the highlight of the day, retold with giggles as the children devoured cake and ice cream. Long after the party ended, Sophie insisted that her balloons were still floating somewhere above, throwing a birthday celebration of their own.

Sweaters That Didn't Fit Anyone

Every December, the Harris family held a big holiday gathering filled with carols, cookies, and plenty of laughter. That year, Aunt Margaret decided to add a special surprise. She spent weeks knitting sweaters for every family member, carefully choosing bright colors and festive patterns. She imagined the family photo with everyone smiling in her handmade creations.

On the evening of the party, she proudly handed out the wrapped packages. "Open them all at once," she instructed, beaming with excitement. The living room filled with the sound of tearing paper as each person pulled out a sweater covered in reindeer, snowflakes, or jingling bells.

At first, everyone oohed and aahed politely. But when they tried them on, the real comedy began. Uncle Frank's sweater was so small it barely reached his elbows, making him look like he had borrowed clothes from a child. Cousin Laura's was enormous, hanging to her knees like a dress. Little Tommy disappeared almost completely inside his, with only his face poking out from the giant collar.

The room erupted with laughter. Aunt Margaret gasped, horrified at first, but soon she joined in. "I must have mixed up the sizes," she admitted, wiping tears from her eyes.

Instead of being disappointed, the family embraced the chaos. They paraded around the living room like runway models, striking silly poses in their ill-fitting sweaters. Someone turned on holiday music, and soon there was a full fashion show complete with applause and laughter.

When it came time for the family photo, no one wanted to change into proper clothes. They squeezed together in their mismatched sweaters, grinning from ear to ear. The picture captured crooked sleeves, stretched collars, and one very happy family.

From that year on, the Holiday Sweater Mishap became a tradition. Aunt Margaret still knitted sweaters, but she purposely made them odd sizes or added outrageous decorations. The family looked forward to it, eager to see what surprise awaited them each December.

The original photo, framed and hanging in the Harris living room, remained the family's favorite holiday memory, a reminder that sometimes the best gifts are the ones that go hilariously wrong.

Carols Sung with Made-Up Lyrics

Every December, a group of neighbors from Oak Street gathered to go caroling. They bundled up in scarves and mittens, carrying lanterns and songbooks, and walked door to door spreading holiday cheer. This year, the group was larger than ever, with children tagging along and even a few pets dressed in festive bows. Spirits were high as they stopped at the first house and launched into "Silent Night."

The opening went smoothly. Their voices blended together, soft and sweet in the frosty evening air. But when they moved on to the next song, things took a turn. Someone forgot the words halfway through, and the group faltered. A few tried humming to fill the gap, while others mumbled nonsense sounds, hoping no one would notice.

At the next verse, the children decided to help by inventing their own lyrics. Instead of traditional lines, they sang about candy canes, snowball fights, and one very mischievous reindeer. The adults tried to keep straight faces, but soon they were laughing too hard to sing.

By the time they reached the third house, the caroling had turned into a comedy show. One neighbor belted out the wrong tune entirely, while another pretended to conduct the group with exaggerated arm movements. The dog barked along, adding its own enthusiastic voice to the performance.

Instead of being disappointed, the homeowners cheered and clapped. "Best carolers we've ever had," one man said, handing out mugs of hot cocoa. Another neighbor insisted they come back next year, promising extra cookies if they brought more funny verses.

The group continued down the street, no longer worried about mistakes. They sang whatever came to mind, mixing real lyrics with silly improvisations. The sound was far from perfect, but it was filled with joy and laughter.

When the night ended, they gathered back at the community hall to warm up. Everyone agreed it had been the most memorable caroling night yet. Someone suggested officially calling themselves "The Forgetful Carolers," and the name stuck.

From then on, whenever the Oak Street carolers appeared, neighbors knew they would be treated to a show that was part music, part comedy, and entirely heartwarming.

The Church Potluck Mystery Dish

The monthly potluck dinner at St. Mary's Church was always a lively event. Long tables filled the hall, covered with casseroles, salads, pies, and every family's favorite recipe. People chatted as they placed their dishes on the buffet line, proud to share their best creations.

Halfway down the table sat a covered bowl that no one seemed to recognize. The lid was slightly crooked, and steam rose from inside, carrying a smell that was hard to place. Curious parishioners lifted the lid, peeked in, and quickly set it back down with puzzled expressions.

"What is it supposed to be?" whispered Mrs. Daniels.

"I think it's soup," said Mr. Harris, though he didn't sound convinced.

When the meal began, everyone eagerly filled their plates, but the mysterious dish remained mostly untouched. A few brave souls spooned small portions onto their plates, examining it closely. The color was unusual, somewhere between orange and green, and the texture looked like a mix of pudding and stew.

The first person to taste it raised an eyebrow. "Interesting," he said carefully. Another took a bite and declared, "It's not bad, just... mysterious." Soon laughter spread through the hall as more people tried it, each offering wild guesses about the ingredients.

"It's carrot casserole with a secret twist," one woman insisted.

"No, no, it's definitely mashed peas with cinnamon," argued another.

A group of teenagers dubbed it "The Alien Dish" and dared each other to eat bigger spoonfuls. To everyone's surprise, it wasn't terrible—just impossible to identify.

Finally, Mrs. Miller, the church secretary, stood up with a grin. "All right, who made the mystery dish? Confess!" The room quieted, then erupted in laughter when shy Mr. Jacobs raised his hand.

"I was trying a new recipe," he admitted. "It was supposed to be pumpkin curry, but I might have mixed up a few spices." The crowd cheered, thanking him for the most entertaining dish of the night. By the end of the meal, the once-ignored bowl was nearly empty, not because people loved it, but because they wanted to join in the joke. From that evening on, the potluck always featured one "mystery dish." It became a beloved tradition, reminding everyone that laughter and curiosity could make even the strangest food taste just right.

Talent Show Gone Off Script

Every summer, the residents of Pinewood Lane organized a small talent show at the community park. Families brought lawn chairs, kids sold lemonade, and neighbors gathered on blankets to cheer for one another. The acts were always lighthearted—piano recitals, magic tricks, and the occasional juggling routine.

This year, Mr. Thompson, who was known more for mowing his lawn in perfect stripes than for any artistic ability, decided to join. He told everyone he would sing a classic tune, and the neighborhood buzzed with curiosity. Nobody had ever heard him sing before.

On the evening of the show, Mr. Thompson stepped nervously onto the stage. He adjusted the microphone, cleared his throat, and nodded as the music began to play. The crowd leaned forward in anticipation.

He opened his mouth, and for the first few lines, everything went smoothly. But then his eyes widened. The lyrics completely vanished from his memory. He stared at the audience, frozen, as the music continued without him.

For a moment, the silence felt heavy. Then, instead of panicking, Mr. Thompson puckered his lips and started to whistle. The tune was surprisingly good, clear and cheerful. The children in the front row giggled, and soon the entire audience began clapping to keep rhythm. Encouraged, he walked across the stage, whistling louder and even adding a playful bow.

The energy shifted instantly. What could have been an embarrassing mistake turned into the highlight of the evening. People whistled along, some even standing up to dance in the grass. By the end of the song, the whole park was cheering, and Mr. Thompson's nerves had completely disappeared.

When the applause finally quieted, the host handed him a ribbon and announced, "Best Improvisation." Mr. Thompson laughed, holding the ribbon high while his neighbors chanted his name.

After the show, several people joked that they wanted to start a whistling club, with Mr. Thompson as president. He went home that night grinning ear to ear, amazed at how forgetting a few words had made him the star of the evening.

From then on, whenever Pinewood Lane held its talent show, the crowd always asked, "Will Mr. Thompson be whistling again?" The surprise had become a tradition, turning a small slip into a cherished neighborhood memory.

When Nobody Agreed on the Rules

Saturday evenings at the Ramirez house were reserved for board games. Friends and family gathered around the big dining table, armed with bowls of popcorn and plenty of good spirits. Monopoly, Scrabble, and card games rotated each week, but no matter which game was chosen, laughter was guaranteed.

One particular evening, they decided to play a new board game that none of them had tried before. The instructions were passed around, but they were printed in tiny letters that seemed more confusing than helpful. Mr. Ramirez attempted to read them aloud, stumbling over long sentences and complicated rules. By the time he finished, no one was any clearer on how the game was supposed to work.

"Let's just start and figure it out as we go," suggested his sister. Everyone agreed, eager to play.

At first, the game moved smoothly enough. But soon questions began to pop up. Could you skip a turn? Was trading allowed? Did a player lose points or gain them when they landed on certain spaces? Every time someone asked, the group paused for a debate.

Opinions flew across the table. One person swore they remembered reading that skipping was allowed. Another insisted it wasn't. Someone suggested making up their own rule to keep things moving. Before long, each turn was less about the game itself and more about arguing over what the rules meant.

The debates grew more dramatic. Players raised their voices in mock seriousness, pointing at the rulebook like lawyers in a courtroom. The children chimed in too, adding outrageous rules such as, "If you roll a six, you have to sing a song." Instead of being annoyed, the adults burst out laughing and agreed to adopt the new ideas.

By the end of the night, the original game had transformed into something entirely different, a mix of official instructions and silly rules invented on the spot. Nobody cared who won or lost. They were too busy laughing at the sight of Uncle Luis standing on one foot because of a made-up penalty or Aunt Maria singing off-key after rolling a six.

When the snacks were gone and the game finally ended, everyone agreed it had been the best game night yet. From then on, the family decided the only true rule was simple: have fun.

Sold by Mistake at the Yard Sale

The annual neighborhood garage sale was in full swing on Maple Avenue. Families lined their driveways with tables covered in old books, mismatched dishes, toys, and forgotten gadgets. Bargain hunters strolled up and down the street, calling out greetings and comparing their finds.

Mrs. Clark had carefully sorted through her attic the week before. She filled boxes with things she no longer needed and proudly set them out on her driveway. Among the items was a small porcelain vase, a family keepsake she actually meant to keep but had accidentally placed in the wrong box.

Early in the morning, Mr. Jenkins from across the street stopped by. He spotted the vase immediately and admired its delicate blue pattern. "How much for this?" he asked. Without realizing her mistake, Mrs. Clark replied, "One dollar." Mr. Jenkins grinned, handed her a coin, and walked away with his treasure.

An hour later, as Mrs. Clark rearranged the table, she gasped. The vase was gone. "Oh no," she muttered, realizing what she had done. She hurried across the street and found Mr. Jenkins showing the vase proudly to his wife.

"I'm afraid I sold that by mistake," Mrs. Clark explained sheepishly. "It wasn't supposed to be part of the sale."

Mr. Jenkins chuckled and said, "Well, I suppose I could sell it back to you... for two dollars." His wife playfully elbowed him, but Mrs. Clark laughed too. She handed him the extra dollar and carried the vase back home, relieved but amused.

Word of the exchange spread quickly through the neighborhood. Soon everyone was teasing Mrs. Clark about her "most expensive mistake." At the end of the day, neighbors joked that Mr. Jenkins had earned the title of "best businessman of the block."

The story of the garage sale bargain mix-up became a favorite at community gatherings. Mrs. Clark kept the vase on her mantle, not just as a keepsake from her family, but also as a reminder of the day she bought her own item back for double the price.

What could have been frustrating turned into a tale of laughter, proving that sometimes the best bargains are the ones that come with a good story.

Laugh Attack at Choir Practice

The church choir gathered every Thursday evening to rehearse in the old hall next to the sanctuary. The air was usually filled with serious concentration as voices blended in hymns and harmonies. But one particular night, practice took a very different turn.

The group had just begun a new piece, a joyful song meant for the upcoming Sunday service. The director tapped her baton and the singers launched into the opening verse. Everything sounded fine until Mr. Bradley, usually reliable with his deep baritone, entered half a beat too early. His booming voice echoed through the room, completely out of sync with the rest of the choir.

At first, the singers tried to carry on. A few glanced at one another, lips twitching. Then Mrs. Davis, standing in the soprano section, let out a small giggle. That was all it took. The entire row of sopranos dissolved into laughter, struggling to hold their notes.

The director raised her hands, trying to restore order, but her own smile betrayed her. Mr. Bradley, realizing what had happened, grinned and shrugged. "Guess I was a little eager," he said, which only fueled more laughter.

Once the giggles started, there was no stopping them. Each attempt to restart the song failed within seconds. Someone would crack a smile, another would snicker, and soon the whole choir was shaking with laughter again. Even the organist, usually the most composed of them all, buried her face in her hands to hide her chuckles.

After several minutes, the director finally gave up on the piece and suggested they take a short break. The singers gathered in small groups, still laughing and wiping tears from their eyes. Instead of frustration, the mistake had filled the room with warmth and camaraderie.

When they finally regrouped, the choir sang better than ever. The laughter had loosened their nerves and lifted their spirits. The joyful energy carried through every note, and by the end of rehearsal the director admitted, "I think tonight's giggles were exactly what we needed."

From then on, the story of the choir practice giggles became part of the group's history. Whenever someone slipped up, instead of embarrassment, it brought smiles and reminded them that music is just as much about joy as it is about perfection.

Who Really Won the Raffle?

The annual town fair was the highlight of summer in Brookfield. Stalls lined the square with homemade pies, jars of jam, and crafts, while children darted between rides and games. The raffle table stood proudly in the center, offering the grand prize of a brand-new bicycle.

All afternoon, people bought tickets and dreamed about winning. As the sun began to set, the crowd gathered for the big announcement. The mayor stepped up to the microphone, holding the raffle drum with dramatic flair. He reached in, pulled out a ticket, and read aloud, "Number six one nine."

Cheers erupted as dozens of people looked down at their tickets. Strangely, more than one hand shot up. Several people shouted, "That's me!" The mayor frowned, glancing at the ticket again. Then someone in the crowd yelled, "You're holding it upside down!"

The mayor flipped the ticket over. Instead of six one nine, the winning number was nine one six. The crowd burst into laughter. People who had already been celebrating groaned good-naturedly, while those who actually had nine one six jumped up with delight.

In the end, only one person held the true winning number, a shy teenager named Lucy. She stepped forward, blushing furiously as the mayor handed her the bicycle. The crowd clapped and cheered, still chuckling about the mix-up.

Rather than feeling embarrassed, the mayor leaned into the joke. "Well, I guess I just doubled the suspense," he said, grinning at the audience. From that point on, he was teased at every community event for needing "raffle reading glasses."

Lucy rode her prize proudly around the fairgrounds while children cheered and adults snapped photos. The mistake made the moment more memorable than anyone had expected.

In the years that followed, the raffle was always announced with extra care. Still, someone in the crowd inevitably shouted, "Don't read it upside down!" and everyone laughed, remembering the year of the great raffle confusion.

What could have been an awkward slip turned into a story retold every summer, a reminder that small mistakes often create the best memories.

Cookies Without Sugar

The Maple Street Book Club met once a month in Mrs. Harper's cozy living room. The group loved discussing novels, but everyone secretly looked forward to the snacks just as much as the books. Homemade treats were a tradition, and each member took turns bringing something special.

One chilly evening, it was Mrs. Carter's turn. She decided to impress the group with her grandmother's famous cookie recipe, a classic that always earned compliments. She measured carefully, mixed the dough, and slid tray after tray into the oven. The smell filled her kitchen, and she felt proud as she arranged the golden cookies on a platter.

When the meeting began, the members settled into their chairs with mugs of tea and slices of cake. Then Mrs. Carter unveiled her cookies. "These are a family favorite," she said confidently, passing the plate around.

The first bites, however, told a different story. Instead of sweet, buttery goodness, the cookies were strangely bland, with a hint of something bitter. Mrs. Thompson frowned politely. Mr. Davis took a second nibble, then raised his eyebrows. Finally, young Emily, the newest member, blurted out, "Did you forget the sugar?"

Mrs. Carter froze. Her mind raced back to the kitchen. She had measured the flour, the eggs, the butter—but in her rush, she had indeed left out the most important ingredient.

For a moment, the room was quiet. Then laughter broke out. Mr. Davis pretended to dunk his cookie in sugar before taking another bite. Mrs. Thompson teased, "Perfect for anyone starting a diet." Even Mrs. Carter joined in, laughing until her cheeks turned red.

The cookies, though nearly inedible, quickly became the star of the night. Members began inventing names for them: "mystery biscuits," "surprise crackers," and "novelty bites." Someone even suggested keeping one in the club's scrapbook as a souvenir.

By the end of the meeting, the cookies were gone—not because anyone truly enjoyed them, but because everyone wanted to share in the joke. Mrs. Carter promised to bring the recipe back the following month, this time with sugar included.

The cookie disaster became one of the book club's favorite stories, retold whenever new members joined. It was proof that sometimes a little mistake can turn a simple evening into a memory filled with laughter.

Spray Battle in the Garden

The community garden was usually a place of peace. Neighbors tended to their plots, humming to themselves as they pulled weeds, watered vegetables, and admired rows of bright flowers. On one hot summer afternoon, however, the calm atmosphere transformed into something far more lively.

Mrs. Lopez was carefully watering her tomatoes when a gust of wind shifted the spray from her hose. Instead of landing on the plants, it splashed straight onto Mr. Brown, who was trimming his roses nearby. His shirt was soaked in seconds.

At first, Mrs. Lopez gasped and apologized. But Mr. Brown, grinning mischievously, picked up his own watering can and tipped it toward her feet. The children playing at the edge of the garden squealed with delight. Within minutes, the first splash had turned into an all-out water battle.

Neighbors joined in one by one. Mrs. Patel grabbed a spray bottle she used for her herbs, while the Johnson twins filled buckets from the garden spigot. Laughter echoed through the rows of vegetables as streams of water crisscrossed the air. Sunlight caught the droplets, making them sparkle like tiny fireworks.

Someone shouted, "Defend the cucumbers!" while another yelled, "Attack the cornfield!" The garden became a battlefield of laughter, with people ducking behind tall sunflowers or using wheelbarrows as shields. Even the usually serious Mr. Clark ended up chasing children with a watering hose, laughing harder than anyone had ever seen him laugh before.

After nearly an hour, everyone was drenched from head to toe. Shoes squelched, hair dripped, and shirts clung tightly in the summer heat. The plants, however, looked fresher than ever, as if they too had enjoyed the fun.

Finally, out of breath, the group collapsed onto benches and overturned buckets, still chuckling. Someone suggested making the water fight an annual tradition, and the idea was met with enthusiastic cheers.

From that day on, the community garden was remembered not only for its vegetables and flowers but also for the legendary afternoon when neighbors discovered that laughter and a little water could bring people closer together than any harvest ever could.

Dancing Contest in the Street

Every summer, the residents of Maple Lane closed off the street for their annual block party. Neighbors brought folding tables piled high with food, children zipped back and forth on bicycles, and music floated through the warm evening air. It was always a highlight of the season, but one particular year stood out above the rest.

As the sun dipped low, the DJ set up his speakers and cranked up the volume. People tapped their feet while munching on hot dogs and chatting. Then the first notes of a lively dance tune burst through the speakers, and a group of kids rushed to the middle of the street, spinning and jumping with boundless energy.

Not to be outdone, a few teenagers joined in, showing off moves they had practiced in front of their mirrors at home. The crowd clapped and whistled. Soon, one of the dads strutted forward, surprising everyone with a moonwalk that looked smoother than expected. The children gasped and cheered, and the mood shifted instantly.

It was no longer just dancing. It was a full-blown dance-off.

Neighbors took turns stepping into the circle, each one trying to outdo the last. Mrs. Robinson twirled her cane like a baton, earning a roar of approval. The Johnson twins performed a perfectly synchronized routine, making the crowd chant their names. Even quiet Mr. Thompson, who had never been seen dancing before, shuffled in with a goofy grin and wild arm flails that had everyone laughing until their sides hurt.

The energy built higher and higher, with the music blasting and the crowd clapping in rhythm. When Grandma Miller stepped into the circle, the party reached its peak. She moved slowly at first, then surprised everyone with a quick spin and a playful kick. The street exploded with cheers.

By the time the music ended, no one could agree on a single winner. The DJ raised his microphone and shouted, "The whole block wins!" The crowd erupted, hugging and laughing as the dancers bowed dramatically.

From that year forward, the block party was never complete without a dance-off. What started as a spontaneous burst of fun became a tradition that united the neighborhood, proving that sometimes the best celebrations are the ones that make everyone a star.

The Couch Stuck in the Doorway

The Ramirez family was finally moving into their new house after weeks of packing boxes and labeling everything carefully. Excitement filled the air as friends and relatives arrived to help. The sun was shining, the truck was loaded, and everyone was eager to settle into the new home.

The first few loads went smoothly. Chairs, lamps, and boxes of dishes made their way through the front door without much trouble. Then came the biggest challenge of the day: the family's enormous living room sofa. It was wide, heavy, and shaped in a way that seemed to resist every doorway it encountered.

Four people grabbed hold and carried it up the front steps. At the entrance, they tilted it one way, then the other, but the sofa refused to fit through. "Angle it more," shouted one helper. "Push harder," yelled another. Sweat poured as they shoved, twisted, and pulled, but the sofa remained firmly stuck halfway through the doorway.

Neighbors passing by stopped to watch the spectacle. Children giggled as the helpers grunted and groaned, wedged tightly between cushions and doorframes. Someone suggested removing the front door entirely, while another joked about cutting the sofa in half.

Finally, exhausted, everyone collapsed onto the lawn, laughing at their failure. For a moment, it seemed the sofa might stay lodged in the doorway forever, serving as a very odd piece of modern art.

Then Grandma Ramirez, who had been quietly supervising with a glass of lemonade, spoke up. "Why not try the back door?" she said matter-of-factly. Everyone looked at each other, stunned they hadn't thought of it earlier.

With renewed determination, they carried the sofa around the house. To their relief, it slid smoothly through the back entrance and into the living room as if it had been waiting for that solution all along.

The family cheered and clapped as the sofa landed in its rightful spot. Though it had taken nearly an hour of sweat and laughter, the victory felt sweet.

From that day on, the tale of the moving day furniture fiasco became a favorite family story. Whenever someone mentioned the sofa, the Ramirez family would smile, remembering the day a stubborn piece of furniture nearly turned moving into a comedy show.

The Midnight Train Song

It was nearly midnight when the last train of the day rattled into the small-town station. The platform was quiet except for a handful of passengers waiting under the dim yellow lights. Among them sat Mrs. Adler, a retired schoolteacher carrying a small suitcase. She tapped her foot gently, humming to herself as she waited.

Across the bench, a young man tuned a battered guitar. His case lay open on the ground, half full of coins collected during the day. He looked nervous, his fingers fumbling over the strings. Mrs. Adler watched for a moment before leaning forward.

"Go on," she said softly. "Play something. We've all got time."

The young man hesitated, then strummed a simple melody. At first it was shaky, but gradually the notes grew steadier, filling the empty platform with music. A mother with two children turned her head, smiling as her little boy began to sway. An older gentleman waiting by the timetable started tapping his cane in rhythm.

Mrs. Adler closed her eyes, letting the tune carry her back to years spent directing school plays and teaching shy students to sing out loud. She surprised herself by joining in, her voice low but sure. The young man's eyes widened, and together they wove melody and harmony into the still night air.

Soon the mother and her children were singing too, their voices small but sweet. Even the gentleman with the cane cleared his throat and added a few gruff notes. Laughter bubbled between verses, and strangers who had never spoken to each other found themselves bound together by song.

When the train finally arrived, none of them moved at first. The music lingered, wrapping the group in a moment too rare to let go quickly. Passengers stepping off the train looked around in surprise, wondering if they had stumbled onto a secret concert.

As the last chord faded, Mrs. Adler patted the young man's arm. "Keep playing," she told him. "You never know who might need to hear it."

He nodded, smiling shyly, and began another tune as she boarded her train.

The story of that midnight train song spread slowly through town, told by those who had been there. For years afterward, whenever someone mentioned the station, people would say, "That was where strangers became a choir for one unforgettable night."

Did These Stories Make You Smile?

Dear Reader,

I truly hope this collection of lighthearted stories brought you a smile or even a laugh or two. Humor has a way of lifting the spirit and turning ordinary moments into memories, and it was my goal to share that joy with you.

Now I'd like to ask for a small favor that could make a big difference. If you found these stories meaningful, funny, or simply enjoyable, would you consider leaving an honest review? Your feedback, whether positive, negative, or somewhere in between, helps other readers know what to expect and guides them in deciding if this book is right for them.

For authors like me, reviews are more than just comments. They are a way to connect with readers, improve future work, and ensure these books reach the people who might need them most.

It takes only a minute, and I'll read every word personally with gratitude.

Thank you for your time, your thoughts, and for sharing this reading journey with me.

Scan to Leave a Review

With appreciation,

Edward

www.ingramcontent.com/pod-product-compliance
Lightning Source LLC
Chambersburg PA
CBHW050749100426
42744CB00012BA/1951